Wake Up Your Body and Brain

Move better, feel younger

SANDRA BRADSHAW

Cover: Painting by Sandra Bradshaw
Author Photo: LeEtta LaFontaine
Illustrator: LeEtta LaFontaine

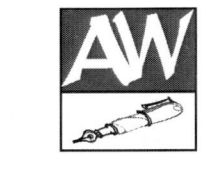

An Artistic Warrior Book

Library and Archives Canada Cataloguing in Publication

Bradshaw, Sandra
    Wake up your body and brain : move better, feel younger / Sandra Bradshaw ; LeEtta LaFontaine, illustrator.

ISBN 978-0-9681694-8-3

    1. Health. 2. Well-being. 3. Mind and body.
I. LaFontaine, LeEtta II. Title.

RA776.B72 2012   613   C2012-907077-7

First Edition
Second Printing

Published by:

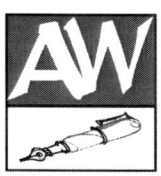

Artistic Warrior Publishing
West Kelowna, BC, Canada
artisticwarrior.com ~ publisher@artisticwarrior.com

Printed in Canada

Table of Contents

Introduction

Body Magic! That's what it felt like the first time I experienced an Awareness Through Movement® lesson by Dr. Moshe Feldenkrais. I was astonished that after a few simple, comfortable movements I was able to notice significant changes in my ability to move effortlessly. That experience catapulted me into a mid-life career change that transformed my life and has allowed me, even as I now proceed through my sixth decade, to move with ease and grace.

Is there really such a thing as body magic? Yes and no. In reality the lessons embody plain old common sense. They help you to discover your ineffective habits and make logical changes that weren't so obvious moments before. However, the real magic lies in the design of the lessons, as each successive instruction taps into the brain's ability to replace existing patterns with more effective ones. Over time, the ease becomes spontaneous so that you don't have to consciously think about what you need to do to keep the benefits you have created.

The nine lessons in this book are a collection of strategies I encourage my students to use on a daily basis. They showcase essential principles that make Feldenkrais lessons effective in increasing ease of movement. Using these lessons you will interrupt the usual patterns of discomfort and feed your brain new experiences that are pleasurable. As a result, new habits will gradually form and you will feel better and more youthful.

Whether you have a chronic condition such as arthritis or fibromyalgia or are simply stiff and sore after a day of computing or vigorous exercise, you will discover that these lessons will boost your capacity to move effortlessly. It is my pleasure to share with you this modest collection of nine lessons that embody the feeling of *body magic* I discovered so many years ago.

About Sandra

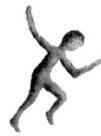 Sandra Bradshaw is a Guild Certified Feldenkrais® Practitioner and former special education teacher. Over the past 30 years she has presented workshops on a variety of topics including yoga, music and movement.

As a Functional Movement Specialist, Sandra's experience using the Feldenkrais Method® has helped her clients improve sports performance in running, golf and equestrian competition, connect with their creative side to improve their dancing, painting and writing and in other cases to increase ease of movement and live pain free lives.

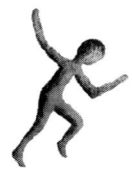

This book is
for everyone who
has the resolution
and tenacity
to improve the quality
of their life no matter
what their circumstances.

Sandra

Acknowledgements

I am grateful for the work of Moshe Feldenkrais. Without his genius I wouldn't have had access to the Feldenkrais Method or to the miracles it has wrought for me and my clients. Special thanks to my friend and publisher, Darcy Nybo who has been after me to write this book for the past five years. I know I would never have attempted it without her nudging. After all is said and done, Darcy was able to spin straw into gold.

My undying gratitude goes to LeEtta LaFontaine, my illustrator. Without her wonderful drawings, this book would never have become a reality. Having LeEtta's support as we tackled this project together was nothing short of a miracle and our shared belief that all things are possible if you stay with it proved to be true.

My two editing angels Michelle McCarthy and Madonna Hamel appeared out of nowhere at just the right moment to give the text the added boost it needed for polish and readability.

Above all, I have to thank my husband Lawrence for putting up with my moods as I wrestled with periods of self-doubt and writer's block and for looking after me so very well for the past 40 plus years.

User's Guide – How to Achieve the Most Benefit from these Lessons

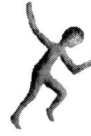 The lessons in this book are designed to boost your capacity to move effortlessly. They are not traditional exercises; they require a different approach. Here are some tips that will help you achieve success.

Note: We all need a reminder now and then so a shorter version of these tips is included in each lesson.

Put aside enough time to read the full lesson. It is important to be familiar with each movement instruction before you do it. Once you are familiar with the lesson and don't have to read all the instructions and explanations the time necessary will decrease.

Reference Movement: Make sure you don't omit this step as it is crucial to your success. Take the time to do the reference movement at the beginning and at the end of the lesson. Habits tend to be transparent so in order to track changes, you must bring your habit to a conscious level. When you have done that, it will be easy to notice changes when you revisit your reference movement at the end of the lesson.

Instructions and illustrations: The instructions are short so you can focus on your movements and how they feel. Once you are familiar with the instructions the illustrations may be enough to remind you what to do.

What Do You Feel: After almost every instruction you will find this heading. I have suggested certain things, but if you don't feel them, that's okay. They are possible observations, so if you feel something entirely different, that's legitimate. The nervous system is subjective, in other words, each person will feel what is unique to him/her.

Choose a Quiet Space: It is important you do these lessons without interruption. The sensations you experience are subtle and if there is a lot going on around you, you may be distracted and not notice the changes.

Make Your Self Comfortable: Remove your shoes so you can feel the floor as a support. Remove any jewelry that might cause distractions including watches, bracelets and necklaces.

Choose a Firm Level Surface: Ideally choose a firm level surface for sitting or lying, such as a kitchen chair or a carpeted floor. If you find this uncomfortable you may do these lessons in an adapted position such as an easy chair or in a bed.

Move Within Your Comfort Zone: Keep your comfort zone at about 50% of your capacity. When you make the movements small and easy you can create a sense of playfulness and curiosity. Your improvement in range and ability will come automatically as you explore and understand your movement patterns.

Make Your Movements Slow and Pleasurable: Learning is achieved when you do what feels good. Your brain and nervous system are designed to respond to two stimuli, pain and pleasure. If a movement feels good your brain will give your body the relax and enjoy command. If a movement feels uncomfortable it will send signals of resistance, which results in continued restrictions and discomfort. With every repetition, look for easier, simpler ways to do the movement.

Use Your Kinesthetic Imagination: If doing a movement causes you pain, do it in your imagination instead. Imagining movements causes the motor neurons in the brain to fire as if you were actually doing the movement. You can do an entire lesson this way and effect measureable physical changes in your body.

Pause and Rest Frequently: You need to be fully present mentally as you do these lessons or you will achieve nothing. The pause obliges your brain to pay attention so each time you initiate a movement it won't become mindless. Pause for at least one breath between each repetition of a movement. Rest completely for a few breaths before you begin a new movement instruction.

Pay Attention to Your Breathing: Don't hold your breath and don't over breathe. Allow your inhalations and exhalations to be unhurried and easy. As you relax into the gentle movements of each lesson your breathing will automatically become more natural.

Note: Once you are familiar with the lessons in this book they can be done almost anywhere and anytime you feel the need to readjust your comfort level.

Enjoy!

Caution: *Thousands of people have benefited from Feldenkrais Awareness Through Movement® lessons; however, we cannot anticipate the needs and/or limitations of individuals. The material contained in these lessons is not intended as a substitute for medical treatment. Consult your local Feldenkrais practitioner or physiotherapist if you have any concerns. Responsibility for the lessons is strictly that of the user.*

Sandra Bradshaw

Lesson #1 – Release Tension from the Fingers

Motion is Lotion

As we age, inactivity contributes to increased stiffness and pain in the joints. This happens because synovial fluid, which lubricates the joints, is only produced when we move. The gentle, pleasurable movements in this lesson stimulate the production of synovial fluid in the finger joints which eases tension and discomfort when using your hands.

This lesson illustrates how only a little movement is required to ease discomfort. Remember, gentle and slow motion is lotion.

Time required to learn lesson
- 15 – 20 minutes

You will need
- A chair without arms and a firm level seat.
- A tennis ball or a ball of similar size. If you don't have a ball, a firmly rolled up sock will work.

Take time to read the full lesson before you do it.

Reference movement – notice how you normally move.

What to do

- Sit towards the front of your chair with your feet flat on the floor a comfortable distance apart.
- Put the tennis ball off to the side for the moment so that you can rest both hands on your thighs, palm facing up.
- Slowly open and close your hands a few times.

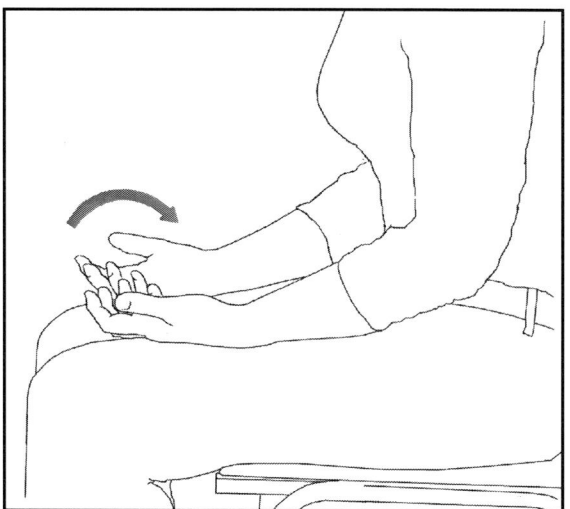 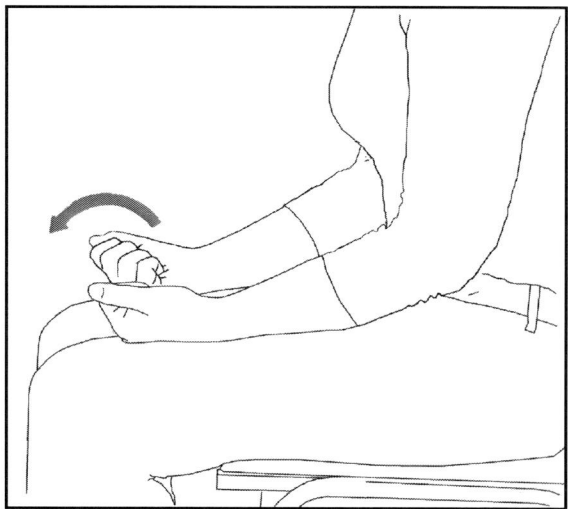

What do you feel

- Does it feel easy to move your fingers or are there some restrictions.
- Do both hands feel the same or is there a difference in the quality of the movement in one hand compared to the other?
- Does one hand feel stronger than the other?

If the movement in one hand feels more restricted than the other, begin with that hand. If there isn't any difference, start with either hand.

You will revisit your reference movement at the end of the lesson.

Sandra Bradshaw

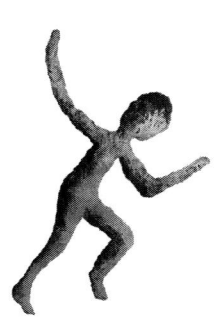

Tips for effortless movement:

Move slowly and make movements pleasurable.

Breathe naturally in an unhurried, easy manner.

Reduce effort to 50% of your capability.

Imagine a movement if doing it causes discomfort or pain.

Repeat each movement 3 or 4 times pausing between repetitions.

Starting Position

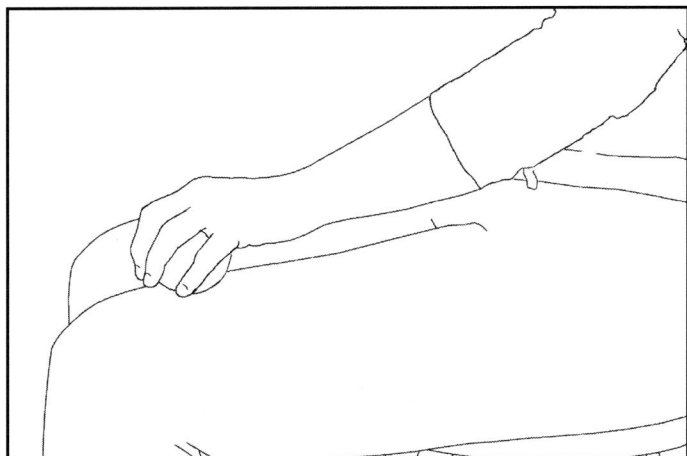

- Put the tennis ball on your thigh and drape your hand over it.
- Let your hand be completely passive with the center of your palm resting on top of the ball.
- Don't grasp the ball, simply let your fingers gently drape over the sides.
- At the same time, allow your whole arm to be relaxed so that you're not holding tension in your shoulder.
- The weight of your whole arm should rest on the ball.

Sometimes when we concentrate we hold our breath. Holding the breath creates tension in the body and movement becomes more difficult. Let your breathing be easy and unhurried as you continue with each movement instruction.

Make sure you are sitting comfortably.

When you create tension, recognize it and learn to release it.

Movement #1

- Grasp the ball tightly.
- Hold this position for a few seconds.
- Release the tight grasp.

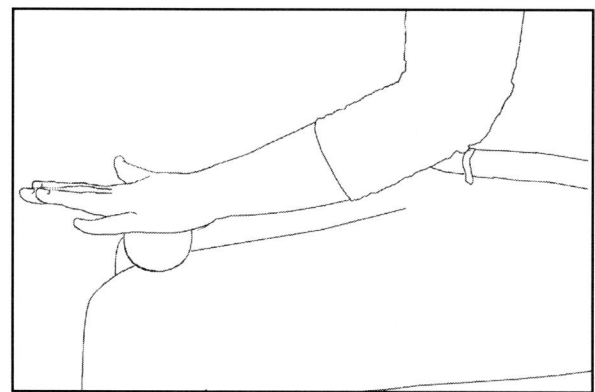

What do you feel

- How do your fingers feel when you tighten your hand around the ball?
- How do your fingers feel when you release the tension?

Movement #2

- Stretch your fingers out making your entire hand flat like a board.
- Hold this position for a few seconds.
- Relax your fingers and allow them to once again rest against the contour of the ball.

What do you feel

- How do your fingers feel when you extended them?
- Do you feel any tension in your hand and arm?
- What happens to the tension when you rest your fingers around the ball?

Rest between each numbered instruction.

Sandra Bradshaw

Repeat each set of instructions 3 or 4 times.

Movement #3

- Let your fingers drape over the ball.
- Lift your shoulder.
- Hold the position for 2 or 3 seconds.
- Release the shoulder and let the weight of your arm rest on the ball.

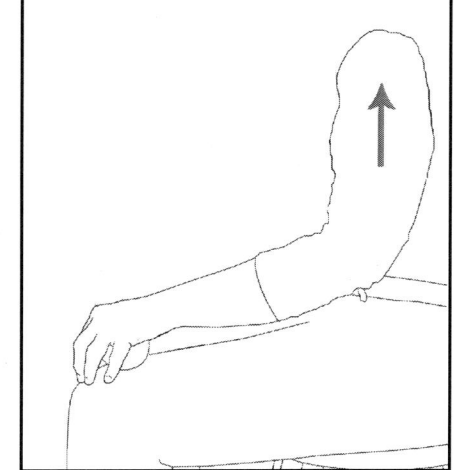

What do you feel

- How does your neck feel when the shoulder is in the lifted position?
- How does it change when you release the shoulder?

For the rest of the lesson relax your arm and hand. Allow fingers to drape over the ball in a relaxed manner.

Movement #4

- Move your whole arm slightly backwards. This tiny movement will allow the ball to roll in the direction of your fingers.
- When you feel a slight change in the pressure of the ball against your fingers, pause, and then roll the ball back to the center of your palm.

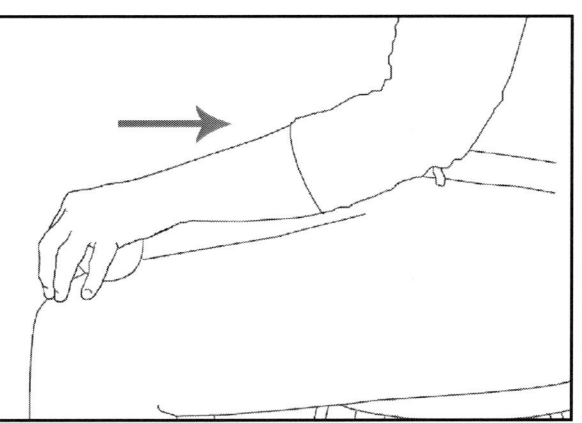

What do you feel

- Do you breathe as you move your hand?

Make the movement easy and relaxed. Reduce your effort.

Movement #5

- Start with the ball in the center of your palm.
- Move your arm slightly backwards until you feel a slight increase in pressure against your thumb (1).
- Move your arm a little forward so the ball returns to the center of your palm.
- Next, roll the ball backwards until you feel a change in pressure against your index finger (2).
- Then, roll the ball back to the center of your palm.
- Continue in the same fashion against the middle finger (3), then the ring finger (4) and finally the little finger (5).

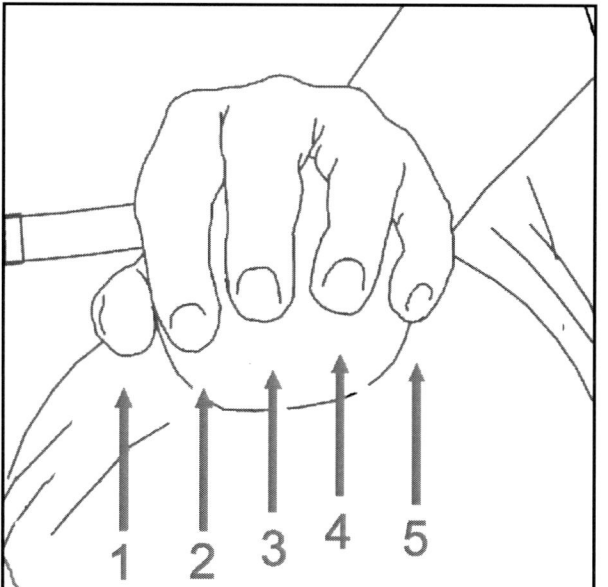

What do you feel

- Notice how your your arm feels.
- Is it relaxed?
- Are your fingers still draped over the ball or are they clutching the ball?

Pause between each initiation of a movement.

Breathe gently. Holding the breath creates added tension.

Movement #6

- Roll the ball in a little circle in the center of your palm in a leisurely way.

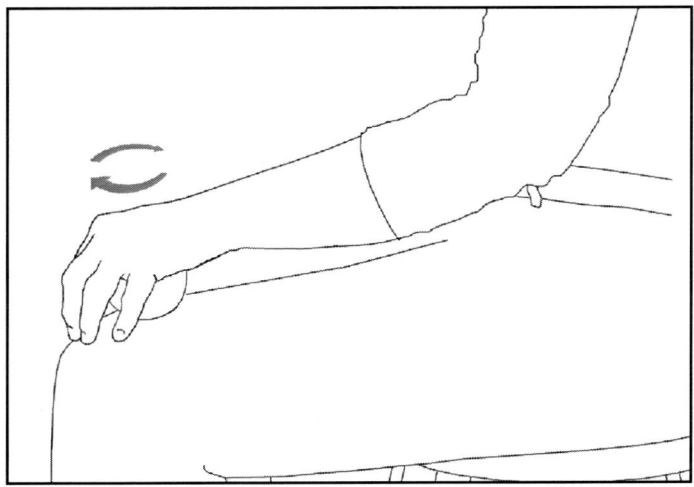

- Allow your shoulder and arm to be relaxed. A soft easy movement in the hand requires a letting go in the shoulder.

- Go a few rounds in one direction, pause, and then go in the other direction.

- Let your hand feel the contour of the ball as it moves.

What do you feel

- Does your shoulder and arm stay relaxed as you move your hand in a circle?

Take time to enjoy the pleasurable sensation you feel. Brain patterns change only when something is done or felt with awareness. The nervous system reacts to pleasure and pain. If something feels pleasurable, it will be noticed and recorded in the brain.

Rest briefly between movements.

Reference movement – notice the changes.

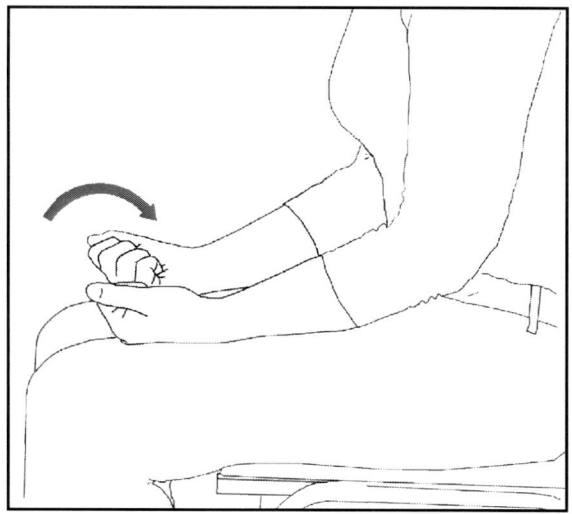 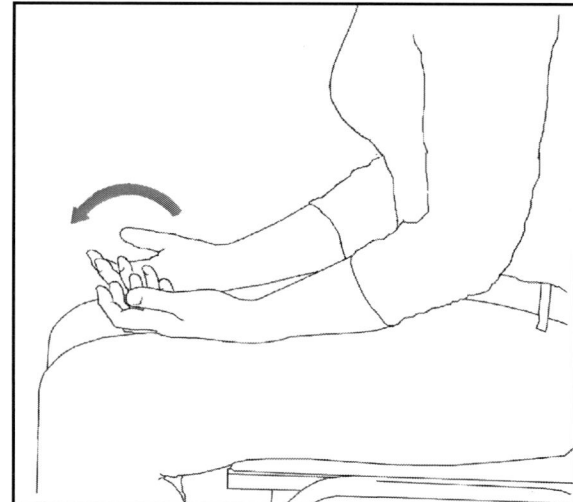

- Put the ball to one side. Rest your hands on your thighs, palms up.
- Open and close the fingers of the hand you are working with.
- Now open and close the fingers of your other hand.
- Open and close both hands together to compare the ability of one hand to the other.

What do you feel
- Did this lesson affect the hand you worked with?
- Notice the difference from the other hand.

Repeat the lesson with the other hand.

Sandra Bradshaw

Something to consider.

For permanent change to occur you need to be aware of your old habits and to recognize what you can do to create a more functional pattern. Moshe Feldenkrais said, "If you don't know what you're doing you can't change your behavior."

Take the time to write notes on your experience with these movements.

Notes

Sandra Bradshaw

Lesson #2 – Look Up with Ease

Using the Imagination to Improve Your Movements

Practice makes perfect. Or does it? Have you ever practiced something repeatedly hoping for improvement only to find that improvement seems to elude you? This lesson challenges you to do something different. It asks your brain to wake up, to imagine movements and to feel what it would be like if you were actually performing them.

For a person with limited range of motion or chronic pain, using the imagination is a pain-free alternative to actually doing movements. You can use this strategy for all the lessons in this book.

Time required to learn lesson
- 20 – 25 minutes

You will need
- A chair without arms and a firm level seat.

Time to read the full lesson before you do it.

Reference movement – notice how you normally move.

What to do

- Sit towards the front of your chair, feet flat on the floor a comfortable distance apart.

- Have your hands resting on your thighs.

- Without pushing yourself or going into discomfort; look up the wall towards the ceiling.

- When you come to the end of your comfortable range stay there.

- Draw an imaginary line from the tip of your nose to the place on the wall where your nose is pointing.

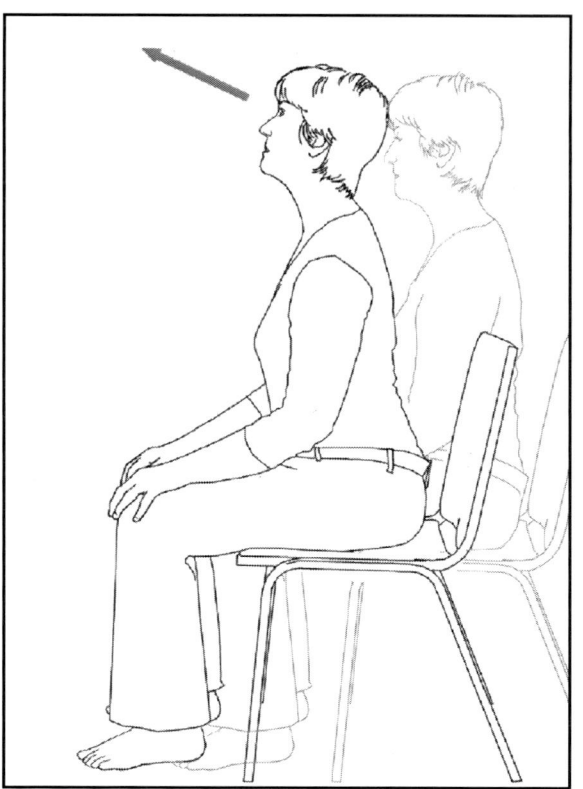

What do you feel

- How far up the wall are you looking? This is your reference point.

Make sure that you remember this reference point. You will come back to it at the end of the lesson to compare your range and comfort. Establishing either a movement reference or a visual reference point will help you to identify changes.

You will revisit your reference movement at the end of the lesson.

Sandra Bradshaw

Effortless movement tips are at the top and bottom of each page.

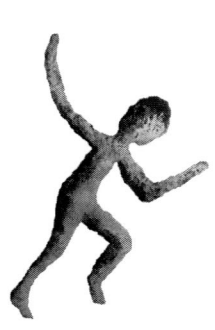

Tips for effortless movement:

Move slowly and make movements pleasurable.

Breathe naturally in an unhurried, easy manner.

Reduce effort to 50% of your capability.

Imagine a movement if doing it causes discomfort or pain.

Repeat each movement 3 or 4 times pausing between repetitions.

Movement #1

- Choose one foot that you will slide back and forth on the floor.
- Look at that foot as you slide it away from you. Do it as if you were trying to feel the surface of the floor through the sole of your foot.
- Go only as far as is comfortable and easy and then return to your starting position.
- Now do it in your imagination.

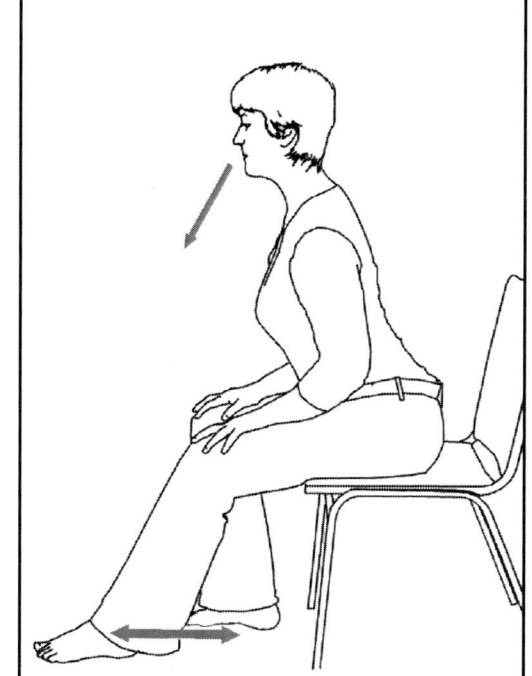

Imagine:

- The feeling of moving the foot.
- How your back moved.
- How your eyes tracked your foot.

What do you feel

- Do you feel your muscles wanting to move as you imagine the movement?

Do each set of movements once. Imagine them 3 or 4 times.

Using the imagination is as effective as doing the movement.

Movement #2

- Continue to look at your foot.
- Round your back and slide your foot away from you.
- Stop moving before it becomes uncomfortable.
- Return to your starting position and stay there.

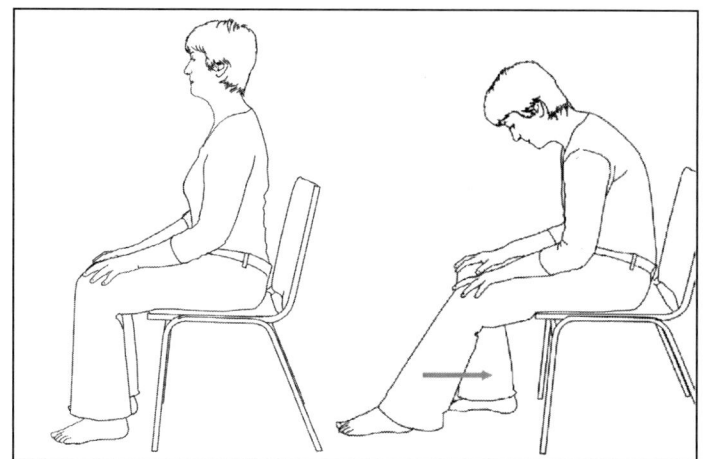

Imagine:

- How your eyes track your foot.
- How your head moves forward as your back rounds.
- How the weight in your pelvis shifts backward as your back rounds and your leg lengthens.

Movement #3

- Continue to look at your foot.
- Arch your back as you slide your foot away from you.
- Return to your starting position and stay there.

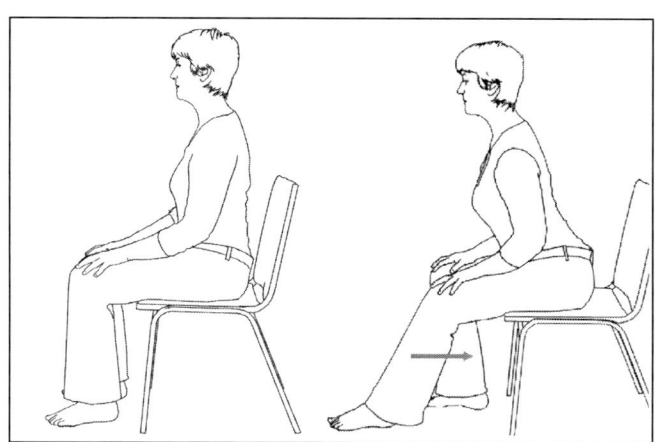

Imagine:

- How your eyes track your foot.
- How your pelvis tips forward when you arch your back.
- How the weight in your pelvis shifts forward as your back arches and your leg lengthens.

Move slowly and never go past the point of comfort.

Remember to breathe as you imagine the movements.

Movement #4

- Continue to look at your foot.
- Round your back and slide your foot away from you.
- Arch as you slide your foot back to its starting position.
- Return to your starting position and stay there.

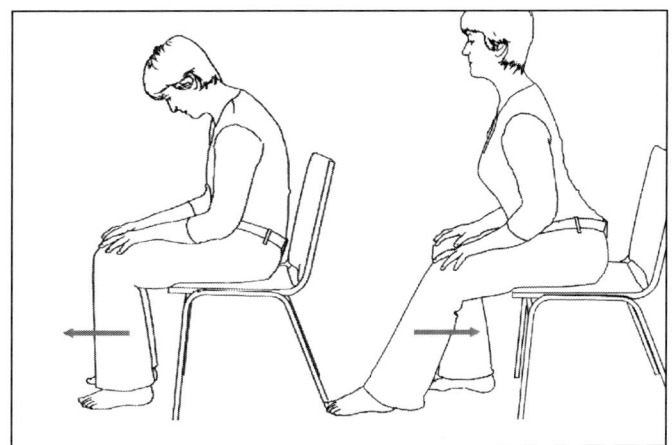

Imagine:

- How your eyes track your foot.
- How your pelvis tips back as you round your back and extend your foot.
- How your pelvis tips forward as you arch and slide your foot back.
- How the feeling in your foot changes as it moves back and forth.

Movement #5

- Continue to look at your foot.
- Arch your back and slide your foot away from you.
- Round your back as your foot returns to its starting position.

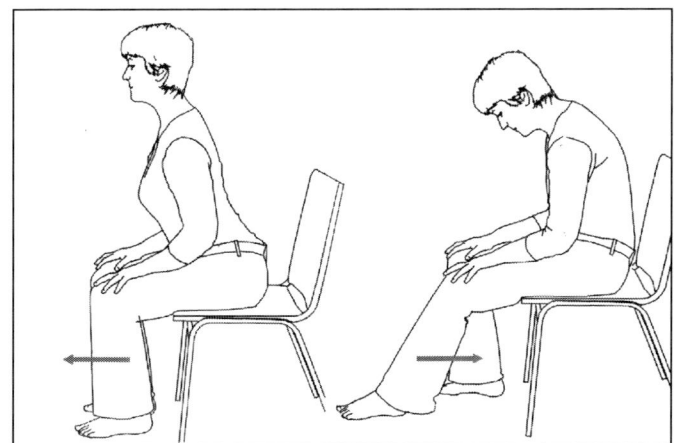

Imagine:

- How your eyes track your foot.
- How your pelvis tips forward as you arch and extend your foot.
- How your pelvis tips back when you round and slide your foot back.
- How the feeling in your foot changes as it moves back and forth.

Try to include physical sensations as you imagine a movement.

Reference movement – notice the changes.

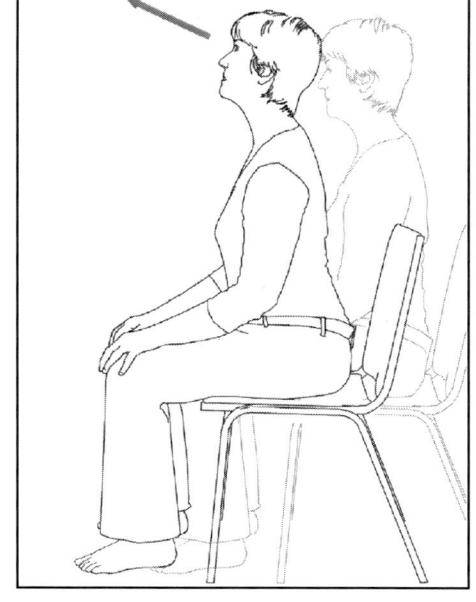

- Sit towards the front of your chair, feet flat on the floor a comfortable distance apart.
- Have your hands resting on your thighs.
- Without pushing yourself or going into discomfort, look up the wall towards the ceiling and when you come to the end of your comfortable range stay there.
- Draw an imaginary line from the tip of your nose to the place on the wall where your nose is pointing.
- Remember where your reference was at the beginning of the lesson.
- Measure the distance between where you are looking now and your old reference point.

What do you feel

- Compare where you are now to your original reference point.
- Do you automatically include more of your body as you execute the movement?

Enjoy what you have created!

Sandra Bradshaw

Something to consider.

The lesson you have just experienced challenges the assumption that you need to physically practice a movement if you wish to improve it. You have learned that using your imagination is as powerful a tool as physical activity.

Although you can do this lesson physically, brain research now shows that imagining movements is as effective as doing them. Your muscles are actually firing even though you aren't executing the movements. This is a technique that elite athletes use to enhance their level of performance.

There is another aspect to this lesson that may puzzle you. Why would looking down at your foot as it moves make a difference in your ability to look up? The brain pays attention to novelty. If you only practice something familiar, the brain goes to auto pilot because there is nothing to learn. When you do novel movements brain activity accelerates as it tries to make sense of new information.

In this lesson all of the movements you do when you look at your foot are also necessary when you look up. When the movements are in an unfamiliar arrangement your brain becomes more alert. With increased awareness the brain has access to more options. A new way of doing the original movement emerges that feels better and is more functional.

Imagination is a powerful tool. Use it.

Notes

Sandra Bradshaw

Lesson #3 – Release Neck Tension with a Soft Gaze

The Importance of Eyes in Movement

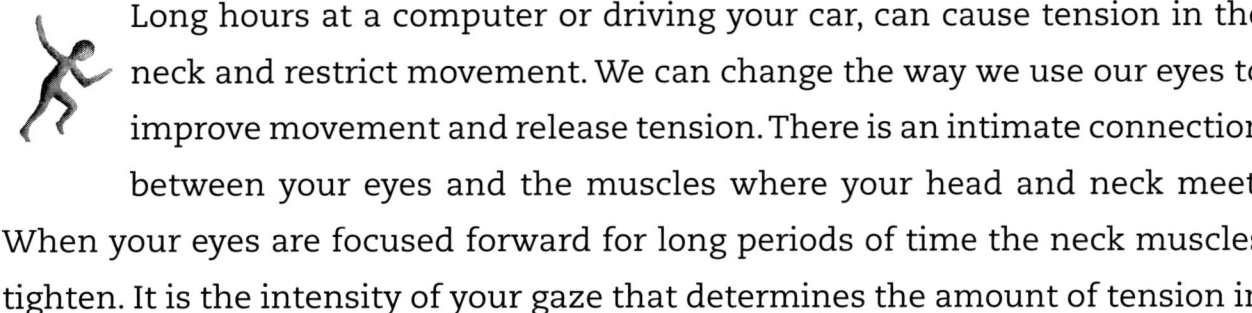 Long hours at a computer or driving your car, can cause tension in the neck and restrict movement. We can change the way we use our eyes to improve movement and release tension. There is an intimate connection between your eyes and the muscles where your head and neck meet. When your eyes are focused forward for long periods of time the neck muscles tighten. It is the intensity of your gaze that determines the amount of tension in the neck.

Learning how to release the muscles behind the eyes and develop a soft gaze will have a profound effect on the ease and range of movement when you turn your head.

Time required to learn lesson
- 20 – 25 minutes

You will need
- A chair without arms and a firm level seat.
- A space on the floor to lie down comfortably.
- A folded towel or small blanket under your head for comfort is optional.

Take time to read the full lesson before you do it.

Reference movement – notice how you normally move.

What to do

- Sit towards the front of your chair.
- Have your feet flat on the floor a comfortable distance apart.
- Rest your hands on your thighs.
- Keep your eyes open as you

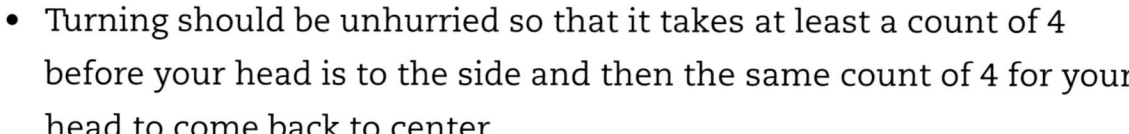

slowly turn your head to one side, and return to center.
- Turn your head to the other side and back to center.
- Turning should be unhurried so that it takes at least a count of 4 before your head is to the side and then the same count of 4 for your head to come back to center.

What do you feel

- Which side is easier to turn to?
- Is there a difference in the quality of the movement on each side?
- What is the range of the turn on one side compared to the other side?

Slow is a relative term and although you may think you are moving slowly you may be moving too quickly to observe what you do. Counting slowly to 4 as you turn will help you to notice the speed of your movement. Once you get the idea of turning slowly you won't need to count. You can then focus your attention on what you are doing.

You will revisit your reference movement at the end of the lesson.

Sandra Bradshaw

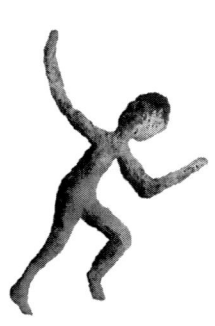

Tips for effortless movement:

Move slowly and make movements pleasurable.

Breathe naturally in an unhurried, easy manner.

Reduce effort to 50% of your capability.

Imagine a movement if doing it causes discomfort or pain.

Repeat each movement 3 or 4 times pausing between repetitions.

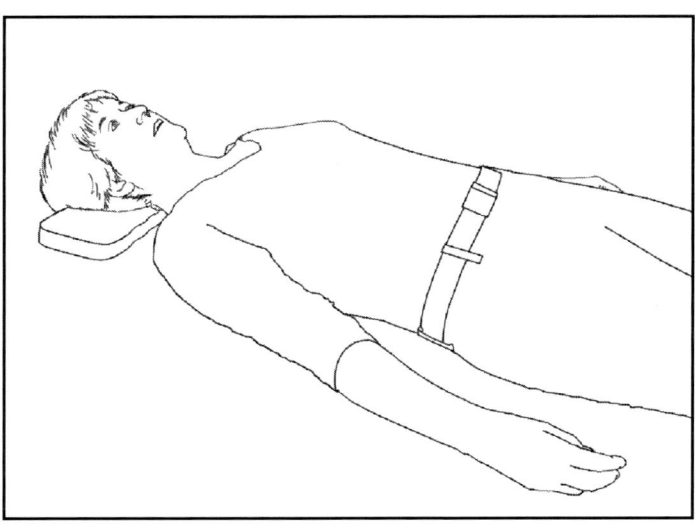

Starting Position

- Lie on the floor with your legs long or knees bent.
- Have your arms resting at your sides.
- Find a spot on the ceiling in the center of your visual field and keep your focus there while you simultaneously do the following movements.

Put something under your head for comfort if necessary.

Read the directions first. Do the following movements simultaneously.

Movement #1
- Pull your eyes forward towards the spot where you have fixed your gaze.
- Lift your head from the floor so the floor does not support your head.
- Clench your jaw slightly so you feel increased pressure on your teeth.
- Hold your breath and make fists with your hands.

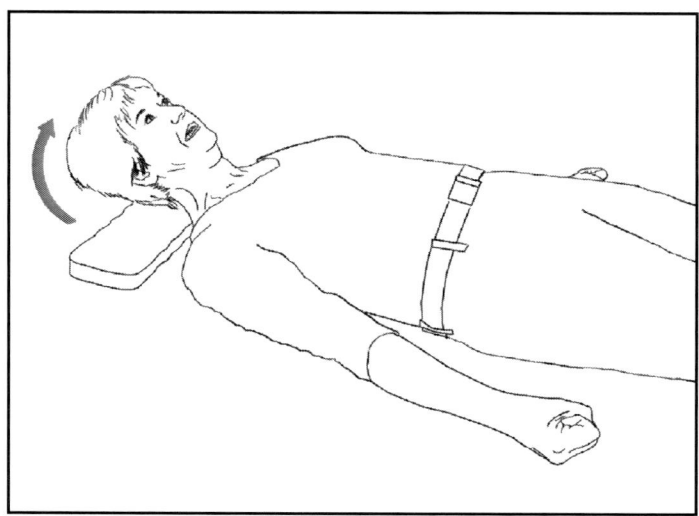

What do you feel
- Take time to notice the tension.
- How does the tension you create affect the rest of your body?

The above direction exaggerates the effects of holding patterns people exhibit in standing and sitting. When you are driving or working at your computer for a long time, you are not aware how holding creates tension until you develop a headache or your neck and shoulder muscles start screaming at you. When you deliberately create the same patterns in an unfamiliar position they feel foreign and uncomfortable.

Hold the position, feel the effects and release.

Sandra Bradshaw

Repeat each set of instructions 3 or 4 times.

Movement #2

- Find a spot on the ceiling in the center of your visual field and keep your focus there.
- Once again, pull your eyes forward towards the spot where you have fixed your gaze.
- Almost lift your head from the floor.
- Clench your jaw slightly so that you feel an increased pressure on your teeth.
- Hold your breath and make fists with your hands.

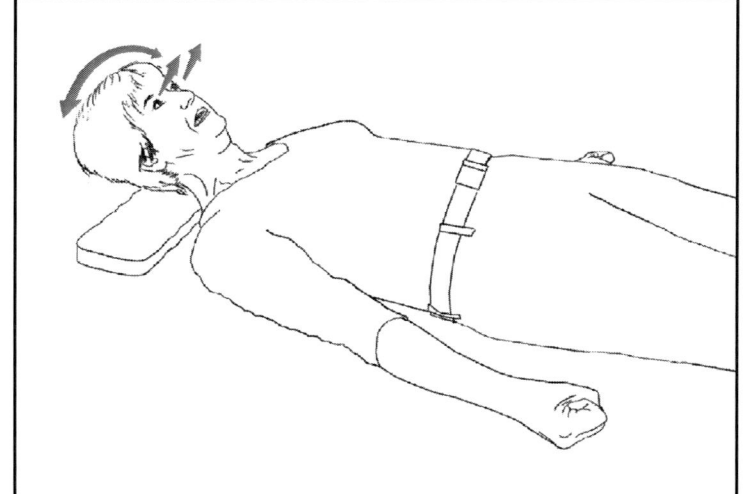

AND

- At the same time turn your head from side to side a few times.

What do you feel

- Notice how the tension affects your range of motion.
- How much effort does it take to turn your head?

Now that you've become aware of some of your tension habits it will be much easier to self-correct when you find yourself going back into old patterns.

Relax & release tension before each repetition.

Rest between each numbered instruction.

Movement #3

Do these movements simultaneously:

- Relax your jaw.
- Allow the floor to support your head.
- Breathe easy and relaxed.
- Expand your peripheral vision. Have an inclusive sense of everything in your visual field.

AND

- At the same time, turn your head from side to side a few times.

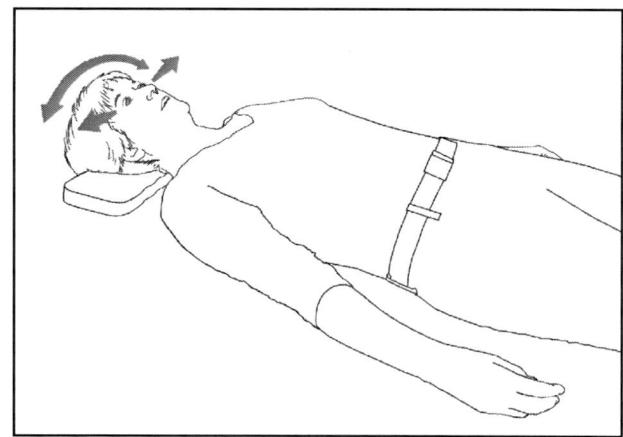

What do you feel

- Notice the difference in the way it feels now compared to when you tightened everything and tried to turn your head.

Movement #4

- Alternate between staring at one spot and the soft generalized gaze which increases your peripheral vision.
- Hold each position of the eyes for about 10 seconds in order to give yourself time to really experience how each gaze feels.

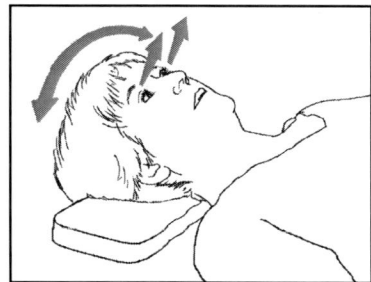
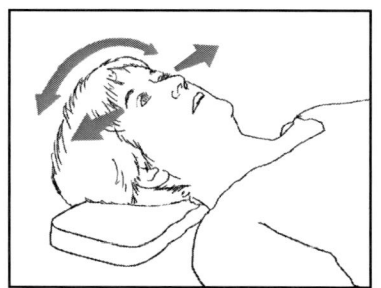

Stop and release all tension before the next repetition.

Remember to breathe.

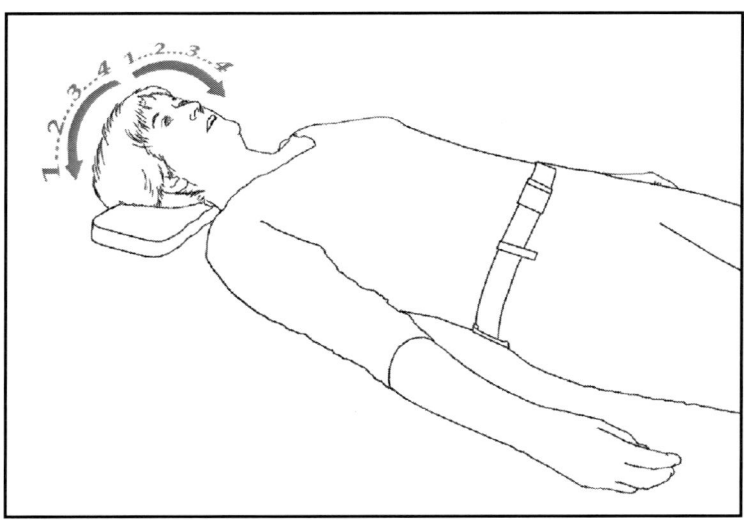

Movement #5

- With a soft gaze slowly turn your head from side to side.
- Take at least 4 counts to turn to the side and 4 counts to come back to center.
- Let your eyes drift in the same direction your head is turning.

What do you feel

- Notice how far can you go without any effort.
- Make note which side is easier to turn to.
- What is your range now?

If you turn more easily to one side than to the other, no amount of stretching or strengthening will balance the range of movement on both sides unless you change your strategy. You need to give your brain experiences of symmetry. By doing less on the easy side you match the amount you can do on the other side. Always defer to the side that does less so it feels easy no matter which side you turn to. Eventually the brain will stop identifying one side as less able and both sides will progress evenly.

The slower you move the more you will notice.

Notice how you can create tension in sitting.

New Starting Position

- Sit towards the front of your chair.
- Have your feet flat on the floor a comfortable distance apart.
- Rest your hands on your thighs.

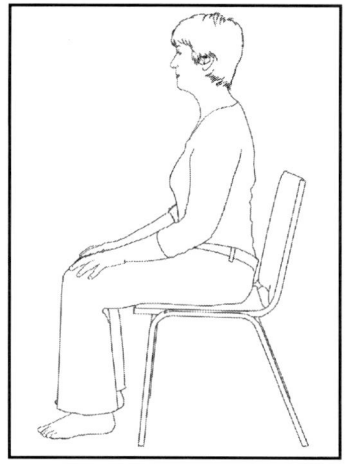

Movement #7

- Stare at something directly in front of you on the wall.
- Pull your head forward toward the spot you are looking at.
- Clench your jaw slightly so that you feel an increased pressure on your teeth.
- Hold your breath and make fists with your hands.
- Hold the tension.

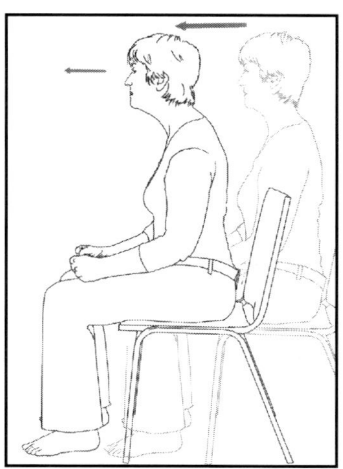

- Turn your head slowly from side to side as you did when you were lying on the floor.

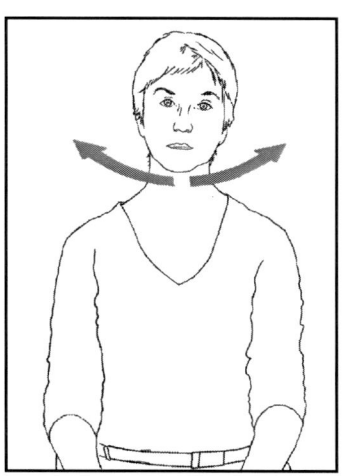

What do you feel

- Where do you feel the tension when you hold yourself in this way?
- Is it easy or difficult to turn your head?

Relax and release tension before each repetition.

Sandra Bradshaw

Reference movement – notice the changes.

Do these movements simultaneously:

- Let your head rest directly on top of your spine.
- Relax your jaw.
- Expand your noticing by increasing your peripheral vision.
- Breathe in an easy and relaxed way.

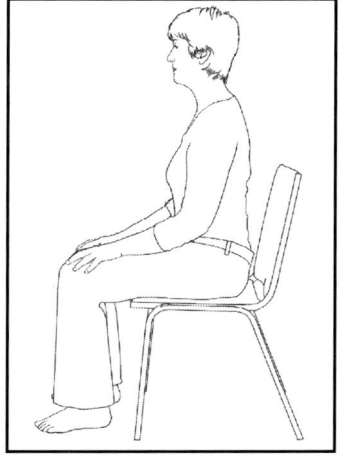

AND

- Turn your head from side to side slowly.

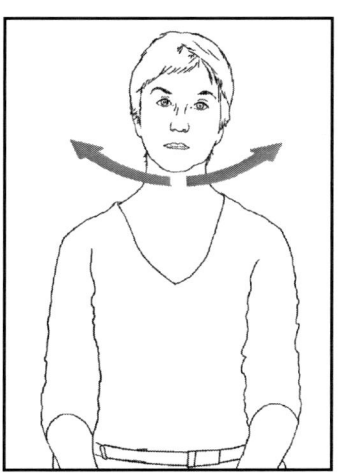

What do you feel

- Notice how this feels different from before when you were staring in front of you and pulling your head forward.

Practice a soft gaze many times during the day and soon it will become an automatic response when you feel tension building in your neck. Learn to use a soft gaze when driving. Your ability to respond in traffic will increase simply because you have a greater global awareness of what's happening around you. Your ability to think while you're on your computer may also change in a positive way. You'll be more relaxed and will be able to channel your energy into more productive pursuits. A soft gaze allows you to look at the life in a gentle way. It takes the strain out of your relationship with the world.

Enjoy the world with a softer gaze!

Notes

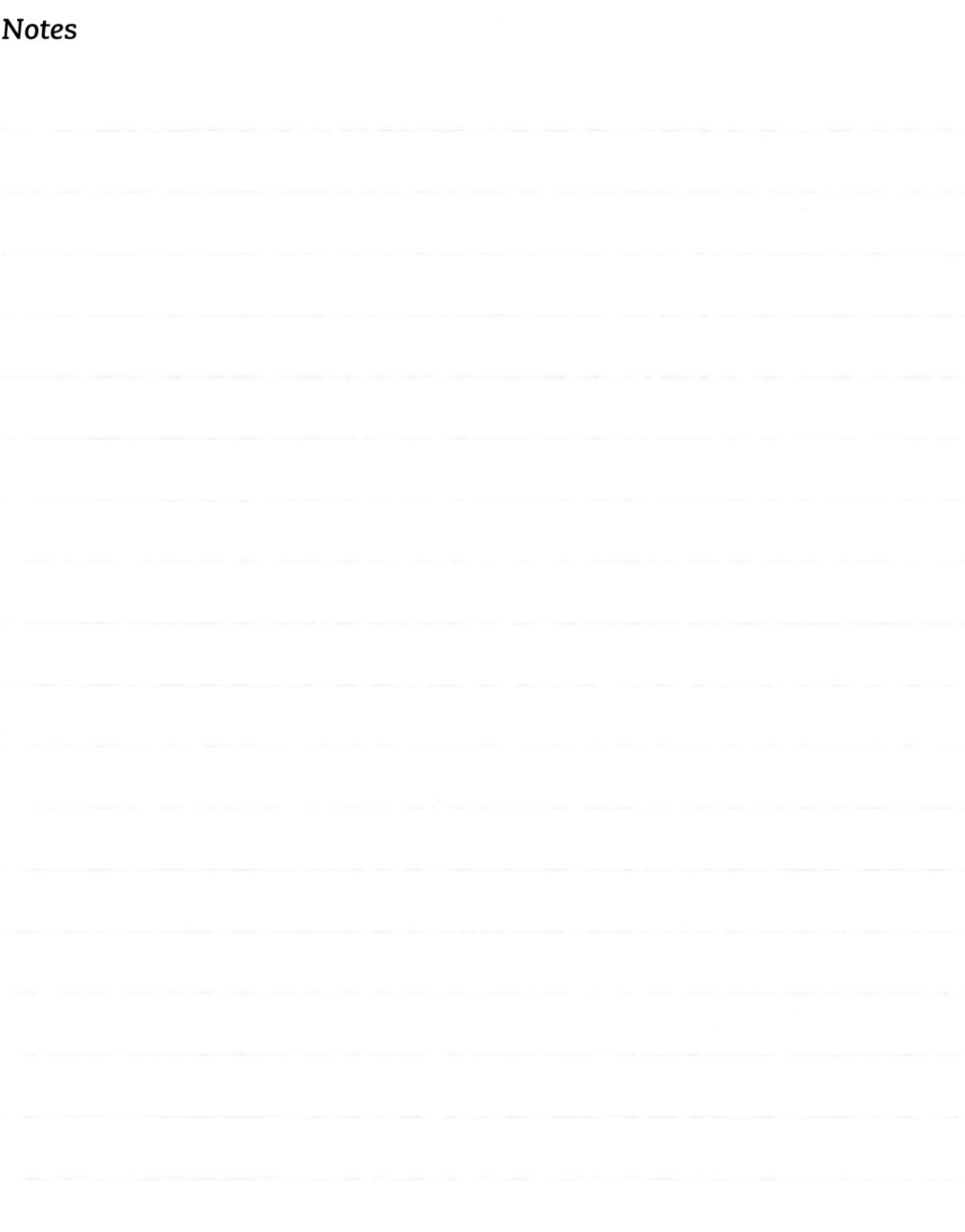

Sandra Bradshaw

Lesson #4 – Release Tension from the Neck

Less is More or Butterfly Kisses

It is commonly believed that physical improvement only comes with a great deal of effort and practice. This lesson illustrates that by doing a few small, gentle movements you will feel a greater difference than you would with many effortful repetitions. I have subtitled this lesson Butterfly Kisses, because when your jaw touches the side of your hand as softly as a butterfly kiss, you will get the best results.

Time required to learn lesson
- 15 – 20 minutes

You will need
- A chair without arms and a firm level seat.

Take time to read the full lesson before you do it.

Reference movement – notice how you normally move.

What to do

- Sit towards the front of your chair.
- Have your feet flat on the floor a comfortable distance apart with your heels directly under your knees.
- Have your hands resting on your thighs.
- Turn slowly to the right and back to center.
- Keep your eyes on the horizon line and let them follow along as you turn.

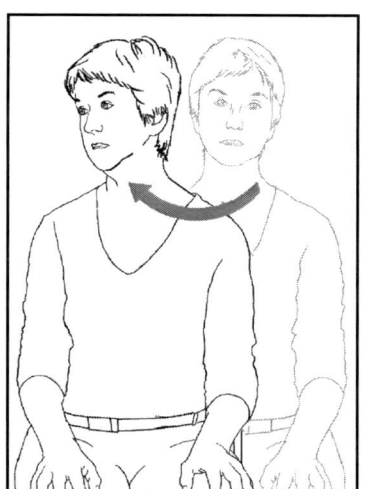

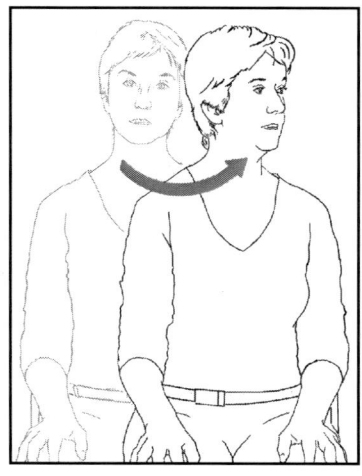

- Do the same movement on the other side.

What do you feel

- Notice if there is a difference in your range of movement from side to side.
- Then note which side has a smoother or easier movement.

If you can turn easily to both sides, begin with either side. If you have a side that is more restricted, the restricted side is the one you will start with.

You will revisit your reference movement at the end of the lesson.

Sandra Bradshaw

Effortless movement tips are at the top and bottom of each page.

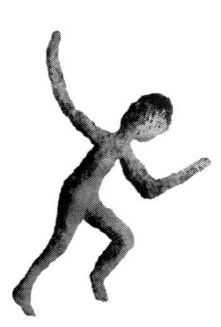

Tips for effortless movement:

Move slowly and make movements pleasurable.

Breathe naturally in an unhurried, easy manner.

Reduce effort to 50% of your capability.

Imagine a movement if doing it causes discomfort or pain.

Repeat each movement 3 or 4 times pausing between repetitions.

Establish a reference point

Note: For this lesson it is important to have a reference point as well as a reference movement which you will use to measure changes.

- Turn slowly to the side you have chosen to work with.
- Make a mental note of the place on the wall where your nose is pointing.
- This is your reference point.
- Return to your starting position.

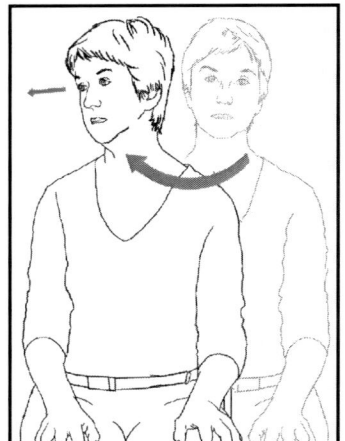

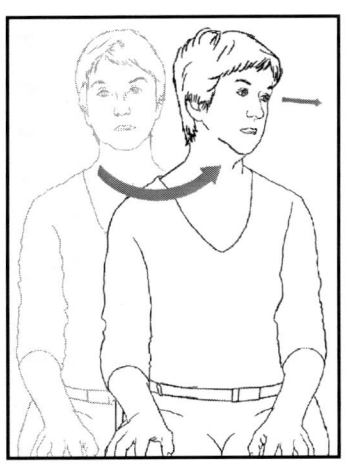

- Turn slowly to the other side.
- Make a mental note of the place on the wall where your nose is pointing.
- This is your other reference point.

Turn only as far as it is easy. Don't strain.

Breathe normally as you turn. Don't hold your breath.

Hand Positions

- If turning to the right felt more restricted, take your left hand and place it on the right side of your neck.

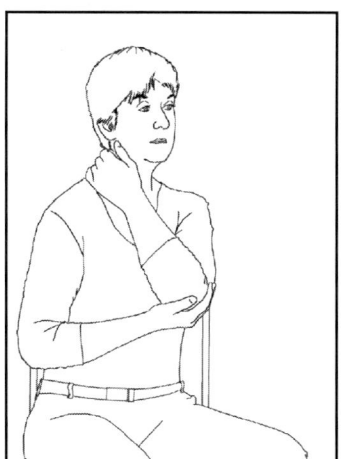

OR

- If turning to the left felt more restricted, take your right hand and place it on the left side of your neck.

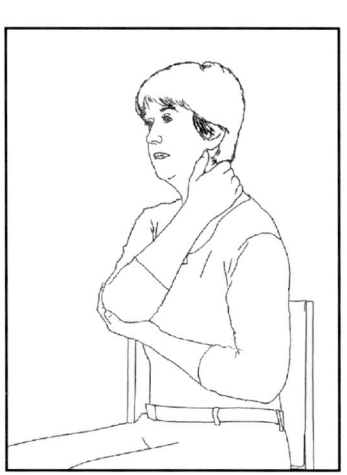

Now

- Keep the thumb and fingers together and gently mold your fingers around the side of your neck.
- The length of your thumb will be just under the line of your jaw and the tip of the thumb will be near your ear lobe.
- Curve your fingers around your neck.
- Support the elbow of that arm with your other hand so that you can keep your shoulder relaxed.

Less is more. Reduce your effort.

Repeat the instructions 3 or 4 times.

Movement

- If your right hand is holding the left side of your neck you will turn your head to the left.

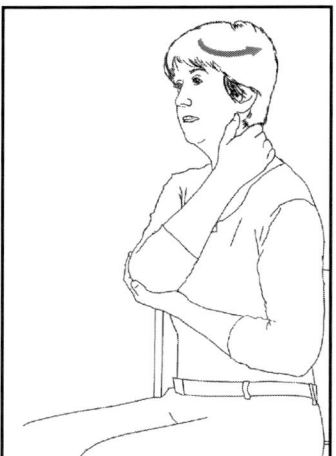

OR

- If your left hand is holding the right side of your neck you will turn your head to the right.
- Keep your arm and shoulders still during the follow instruction.

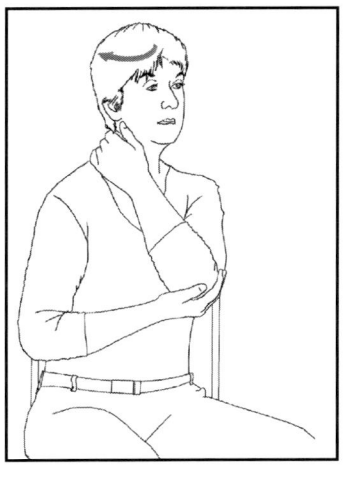

Now

- Turn your head towards the thumb that is under your jaw. Make sure that you are turning and not leaning your ear towards your shoulder.
- Move slowly so that you are aware of the increasing pressure of the jaw against your thumb.
- As soon as you feel a slight change in the pressure against your thumb, stop turning, pause and then return to center.

Note: The pressure of your jaw against your thumb should be soft and gentle. Barely turn your head towards your hand at all. It may seem strange that such a small movement can produce any change, but when you are working with the brain and the nervous system, less is definitely more.

Breathe gently. Holding the breath creates added tension.

Reference movement – notice the changes.

- Release the hand from your neck.

Now

- If your right hand was holding the left side of your neck, turn to the left.
- If your left hand was holding the right side of your neck, turn to the right.

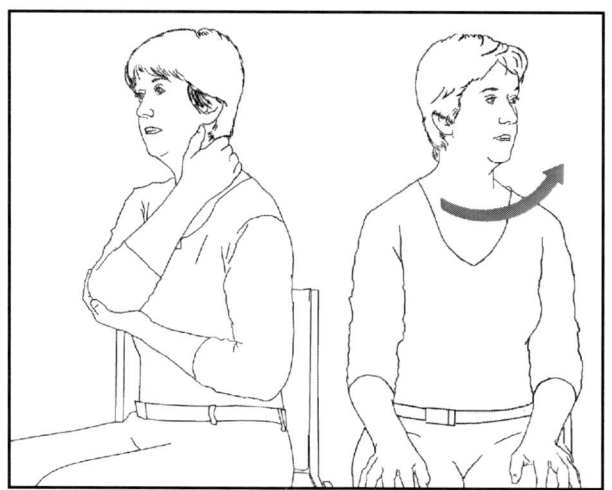 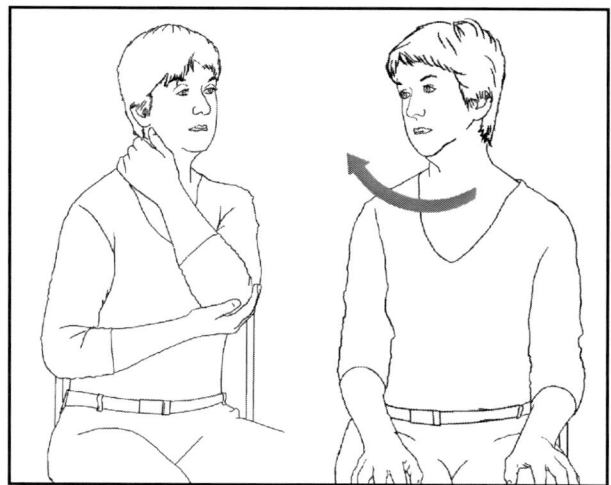

What do you feel

- Note if you can turn farther on the side that you just worked with.
- Has the quality of the movement improved on that side?
- Now turn to the other side and note how it is different from the side you worked with.

Repeat the lesson on the other side.

Sandra Bradshaw

Something to consider.

A wise man once said, "There are a hundred steps between step one and step two."

As you go through these lessons and the small changes accumulate, they will develop into functional adaptations that will enrich the quality of your life. Your brain is designed to accept small, easy, pain-free modifications to movements. Given the opportunity to experience these subtle shifts and the time to integrate them into your habitual patterns, your brain will always choose what feels good and what is functional. Adopt an attitude of celebration.

Celebrate each small success you achieve and your body will thank you!

Enjoy the changes that you have created!

Notes

Sandra Bradshaw

Lesson #5 – Release Tight ShoulderMuscles

An Easy Solution to a Chronic Problem

Chronically tight muscles become more irritated as the day wears on. Often when you finally have time to sit down and relax, your muscles are burning or throbbing. Why does this happen? If a muscle is chronically tight and won't let go, it continues to burn energy causing a buildup of lactic acid. In this contracted state, the circulation is inhibited and the blood can't do its job of flushing out the lactic acid. You are left with a muscle that constantly feels painful. This lesson will show you how to relieve chronic tension and discomfort in the neck and shoulder muscles.

The same principles apply to chronically tight muscles anywhere in the body.

Time required to learn lesson
- 20 – 25 minutes

You will need
- A mirror large enough to see your head and shoulders.
- A chair without arms and a firm level seat.
- A t-shirt with a wide neck so you have direct access to your shoulder.

Take time to read the full lesson before you do it.

Reference position – notice what you do.

What to do

- Look at yourself in a mirror and notice if your shoulders are level or if one is higher than the other.

Choose one of the following options

- If one shoulder is positioned higher than the other. you will work with the higher shoulder for the rest of the lesson.

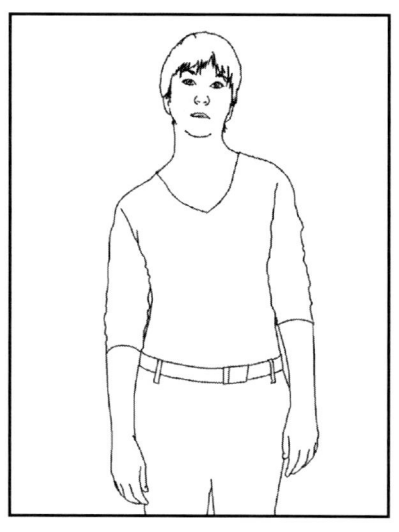 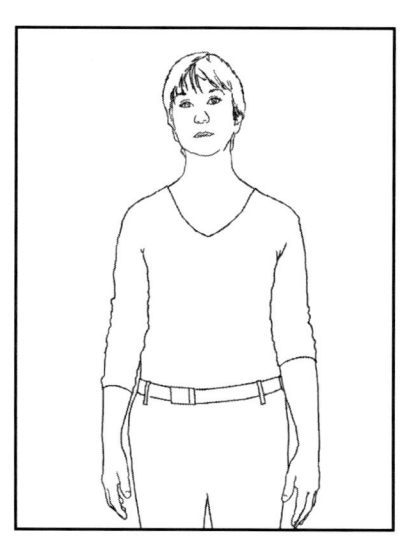 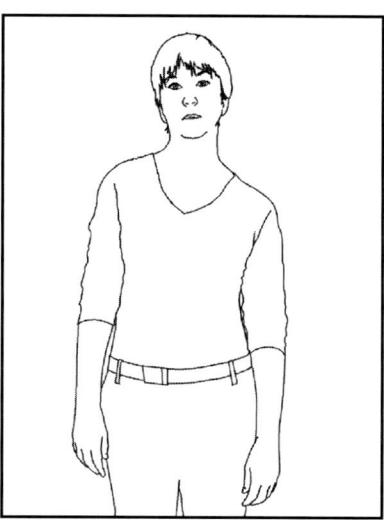

- If your shoulders look level perhaps one feels tighter than the other. Work with that shoulder.

It's easy to see as well as feel tension in your shoulders. Tight muscles lift the shoulders higher than they would be when at rest.

You will revisit your reference position at the end of the lesson.

Sandra Bradshaw

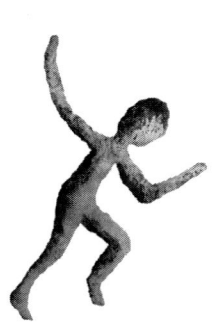

Tips for effortless movement:

Move slowly and make movements pleasurable.

Breathe naturally in an unhurried, easy manner.

Reduce effort to 50% of your capability.

Imagine a movement if doing it causes discomfort or pain.

Repeat each movement 3 or 4 times pausing between repetitions.

Movement #1

- Practice turning slowly on the side you have chosen.
- Take at least 4 counts to turn to the side and then the same count of 4 as you bring your head back to center.
- Keep your eyes on the horizon line and let them follow along as you turn.

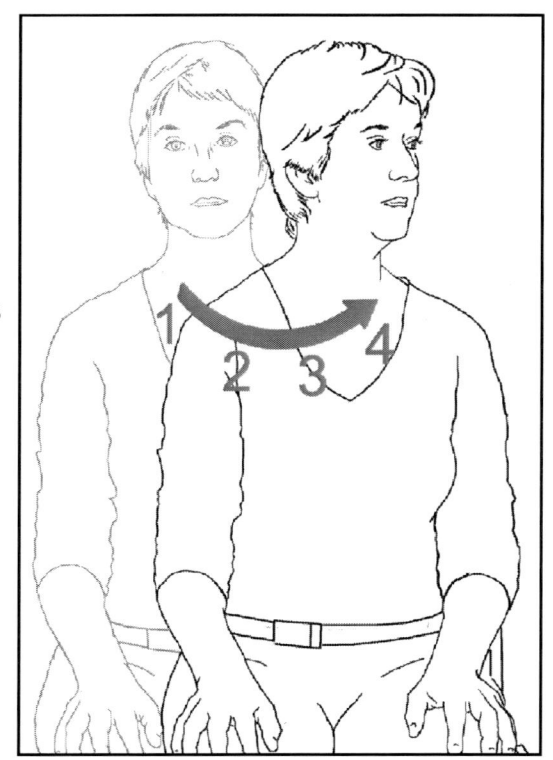

When you hurry movements it is difficult to notice subtle changes. In this case slow down so that you can feel how far you can turn before you have to use effort to continue. When you repeat the movement stay below the point of effort. Your brain will make any changes to the muscles necessary for ease of movement as the lesson progresses.

Take your time. Treat yourself lovingly.

Note: These directions are for the right side of the neck. If you have chosen to work with the left side, switch the lefts and rights in the instructions according to your needs.

Starting Position

- Place left hand directly onto your shoulder with skin to skin contact.
- Support your elbow with your other hand.

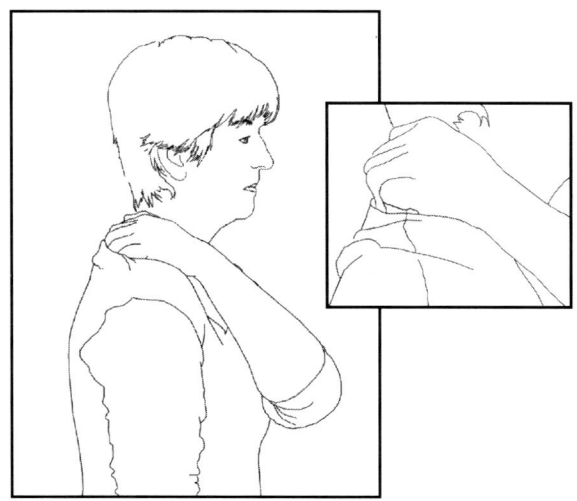
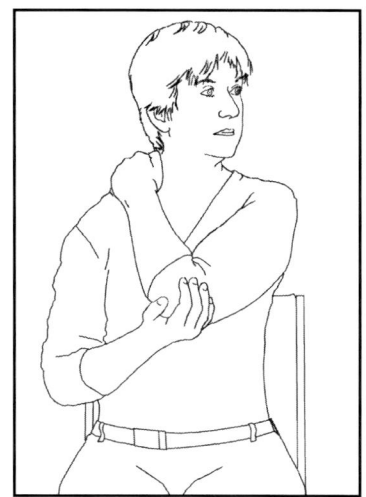

Movement #2

- Gently massage along the shoulder. Start at the outside tip and work your way in towards your neck and then back out again.
- Take pleasure in the slow release of the hand on the muscle.

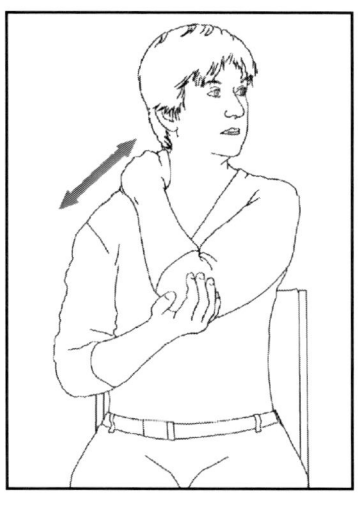

Don't hurry! Take time to enjoy the sensations you feel.

Lift and hold the trapezius muscle firmly and gently.

Refine the Starting Position
- Place your left hand half way between the tip of the right shoulder and your neck, stop there and feel muscle tissue. This is the top of your trapezius muscle.
- The heel of your hand is to the front just above your collar bone and the fingers point down towards your shoulder blade.
- Grasp the trapezius by sandwiching the muscle between your fingers and the heel of your hand.
- If the muscle is tight it won't lift far but you should still feel the layers of skin lift slightly. Release. Let your hand rest there for a moment.
- Lift the trapezius muscle again and hold it.

Movement #4
- With the trapezius lifted, slowly turn your head a little away from your hand.
- Return to center.
- On the final repetition, bring your head back to center.
- Slowly release your hand, lower it to your lap.

What do you feel
- You may feel a slight pull as your head turns away from your hand and a release when your head comes back to center.

Repeat the instructions 3 or 4 times.

Reference position – notice the changes.

- Go and look in the mirror again and notice if the height of your shoulders is more symmetrical.

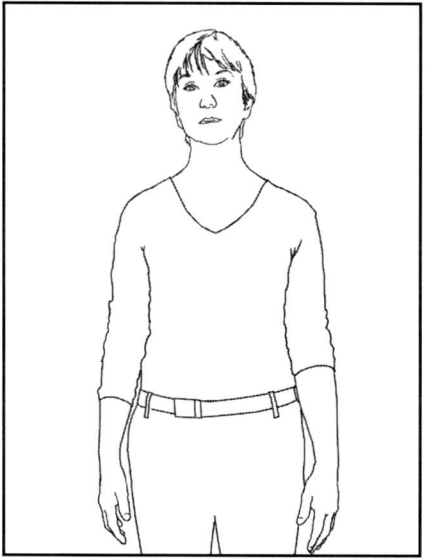

- Turn to the side you were holding. Notice if the quality of the movement has changed.
- Notice if your range of movement has increased.
- Turn to the other side and notice the difference.

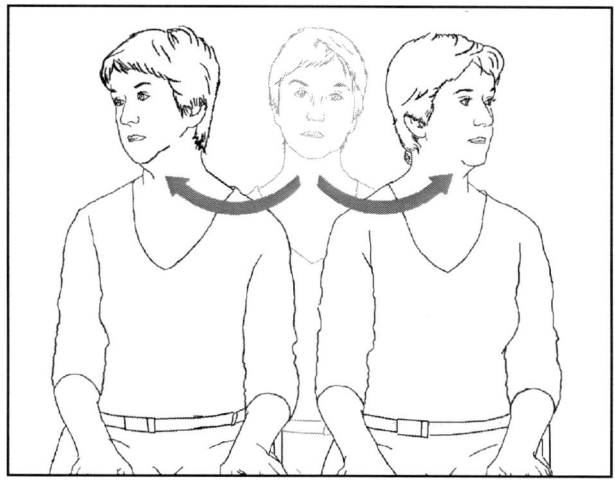

You may find the shoulder you considered to be tighter (or more lifted) feels better than the other shoulder. If this is the case, repeat the lesson on the other side.

Repeat the lesson any time your shoulders feel tight.

Sandra Bradshaw

Something to consider.

To stay comfortable in your body you must pay attention to the signals from your brain.

Your brain works to keep you out of harm's way and to maintain a state of balance for optimal functioning. When things go awry, the only way your brain can get your attention is by creating discomfort and pain.

When you notice these signals and you have the knowledge to bring the body back into balance, the brain will automatically stop producing discomfort and pain.

You can use this strategy to relieve discomfort whenever you feel your shoulders tighten.

Enjoy the changes you have created!

Notes

Sandra Bradshaw

Lesson #6 – Easy Turning

Integration of the Parts Improves the Whole

Do you know what you do when you turn? What parts of yourself are involved in the action? Are you aware of the role your breathing plays in your range of movement? How your pelvis and legs contribute to the ease of the rotation? How your eyes support or inhibit the entire process?

Moshe Feldenkrais said, "If you know what you're doing, you can do what you want."

This lesson will help you to learn what you habitually do when you turn. You will feel the difference when your brain organizes all the parts of yourself in a new, more functional way.

Time required to learn lesson
- 20 – 25 minutes

You will need
- A chair without arms and a firm level seat.

Take time to read the full lesson before you do it.

Reference movement – notice how you normally move.

What to do

- Sit towards the front of your chair.
- Have your feet flat on the floor a comfortable distance apart.
- Rest your hands on your thighs.
- Slowly turn to one side and back to center.
- Repeat this movement a few times and without changing anything.

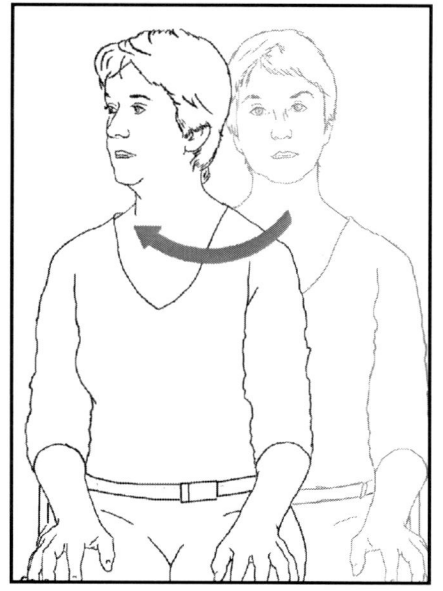

What do you feel

- Notice if you move your shoulders and torso.
- Does anything else move?
- Are you breathing?

What to do

- Now turn to the other side, then back to the center a few times.
- Don't change what you do, simply notice your habit.

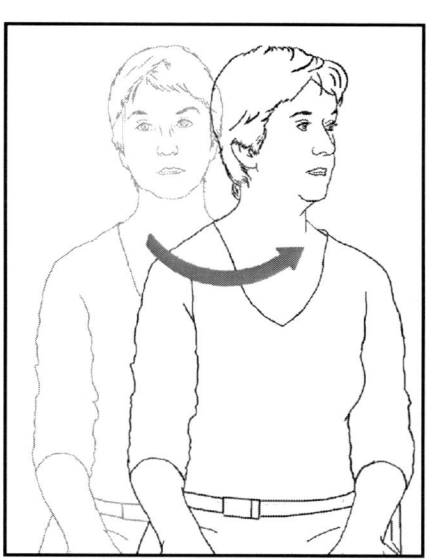

What do you feel

- Compare your range to the first side.
- Is it the same or different?
- Note which side was easier.

You will revisit your reference movement at the end of the lesson.

Sandra Bradshaw

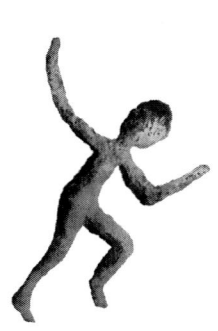

Tips for effortless movement:

Move slowly and make movements pleasurable.

Breathe naturally in an unhurried, easy manner.

Reduce effort to 50% of your capability.

Imagine a movement if doing it causes discomfort or pain.

Repeat each movement 3 or 4 times pausing between repetitions.

Find your reference points

- Slowly turn to the first side.
- Stop before you feel a strain in your neck or shoulders and stay there.
- Look at the spot on the wall where your nose is pointing.
- This is your reference point; make a mental note of this spot.
- Return to center.

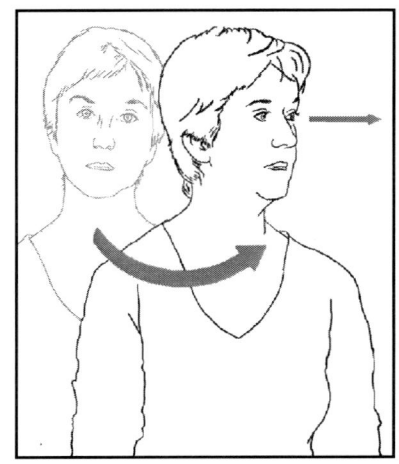

- Now find your reference point on the other side.
- Turn slowly and stop before you feel a strain in your neck and shoulders.
- Make a mental note of this point.

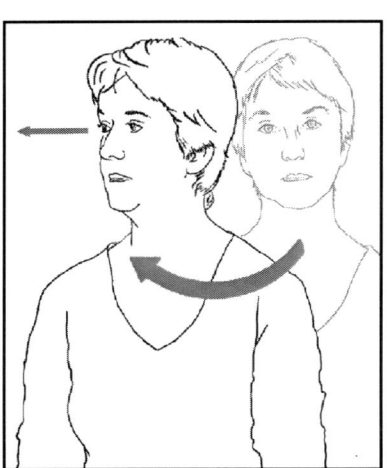

Note: We'll come back to these two points at the end of the lesson.

Don't force the movement. Only turn as far as is easy.

Repeat each numbered set of movements 3 or 4 times.

Starting Position

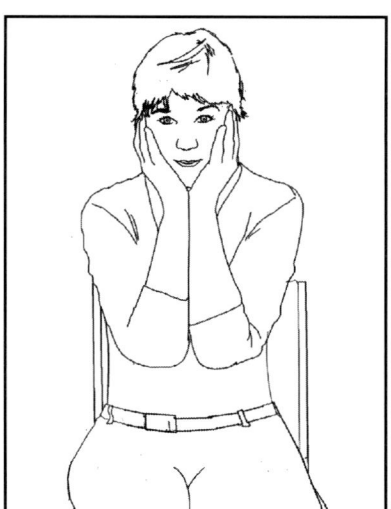

- Bring the heels of your hands together.
- Place your chin in your hands.
- Wrap your palms around your jaw with the tips of the fingers on or near your temples.
- Let your arms rest quietly on or close to your chest.
- Imagine your entire upper body is glued together (in a relaxed manner).
- It is important to maintain the configuration though out the lesson, so the upper body moves as a unit.

Movement #1

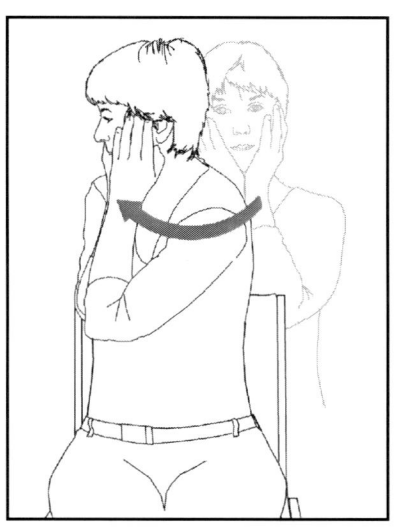

- Slowly turn to the right and back to the center a few times.
- When you turn to the side, notice where the movement is easy.
- When you start to feel a slight pull, stop. Don't go any farther.
- The next few times you do the movement stay in the range where it is easy.

Pause between each initiation of the movement.

Sandra Bradshaw

Movement #2

- Turn to the right again.
- Allow your lower back and pelvis to move with the upper body.

What do you feel

- Notice if the range of movement changed.
- Did the quality of the movement change?
- Note if it is easier to turn now.

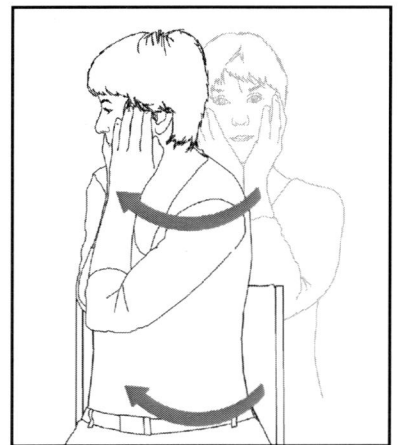

Movement #3

- Continue the same movement of turning to the right.
- This time as you turn your upper body and pelvis, move your knees a little to the same side as the turning.

What do you feel

- Note if the quality of movement improved.
- When you move more of yourself does it change the range of motion?

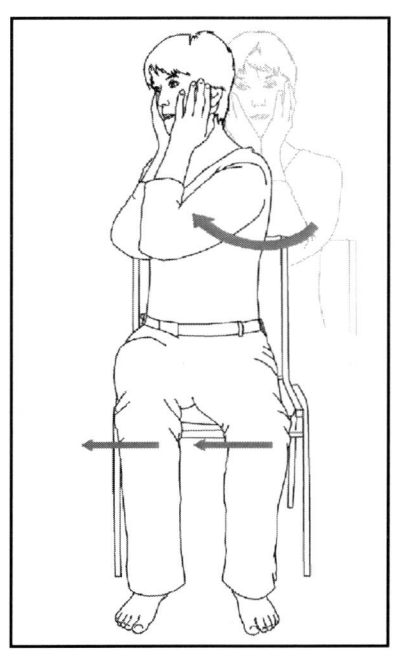

Keep your effort at 50% of what you can do.

Notice if your habits help or hinder the movement.

Note: The next two instructions demonstrate how habits can inhibit range and cause discomfort when performing an action. When you change something as simple as your breathing pattern it can make all the difference between ease and effort.

What is your habit?

- Cradle your chin in your hands and turn to the right and back a few times and notice how you breathe.
- Do you breathe in or breathe out when you turn?

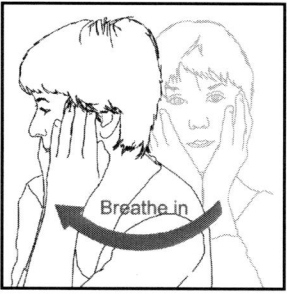

Movement #4

- As you turn slowly to the right, breathe in.
- Breathe out as you come back to center.
- Repeat this breathing pattern several times noting the range and ease of the movement.

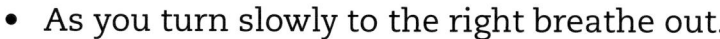

- As you turn slowly to the right breathe out.
- Breathe in as you come back to center.
- Repeat this breathing pattern a few times.

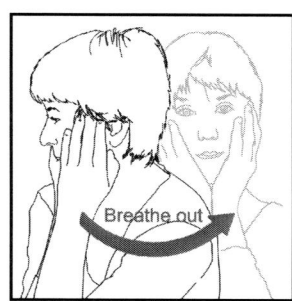

When you breathe in as you turn to the side, you create tension in your body and movement becomes more difficult. Although it may feel unnatural, breathing out when you turn makes the movement easier. For the rest of the lesson, breathe out as you turn to the side and breathe in as you return to your starting position.

Which movements improve your range & ease in turning?

Sandra Bradshaw

Do you move your eyes or keep them fixed when you turn?

What is your habit?

- Cradle your chin in your hands and turn to one side and back a few times.
- Do your eyes stay fixed in one spot?
- Do your eyes move with your head?

Movement #5

- Keep your eyes looking forward as you turn the rest of yourself to the right.

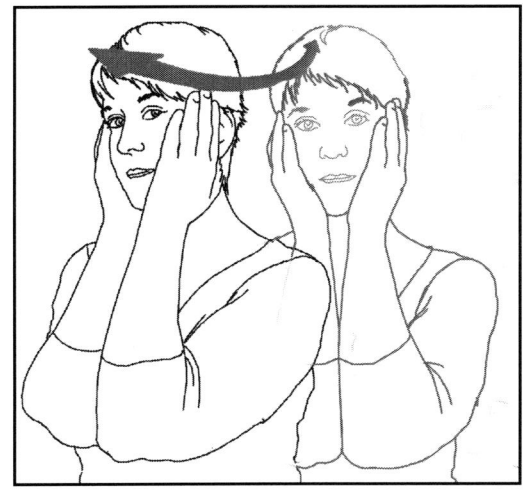

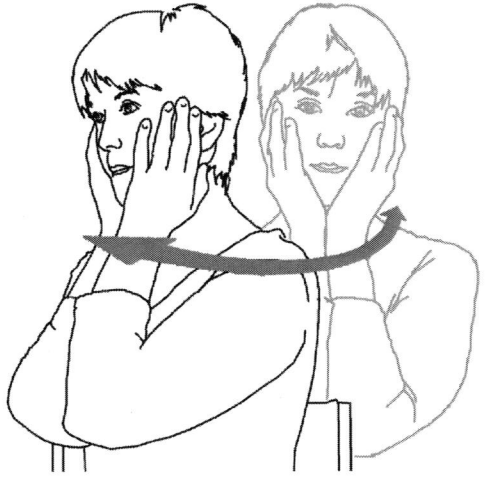

- Let your eyeses move with the arms and head.
- Move slowly as you turn.

What do you feel

- Note if it affects your range of motion when you fix your eyes on one spot.
- Does keeping your eyes fixed change the amount of effort you need to do the movement?
- Does moving your eyes with your body changes the quality of the turn?

Repeat each instruction 3 or 4 times.

Integrating the parts. Putting it all together.

When all the parts of the body are integrated into the movement, the brain spreads the workload through the entire system. This is the key to easier movement. So far you have experienced a variety of specific movements. When combined, they will make the final movement easier and improve your ability to turn.

Note: In this instruction you will put into practice everything you have learned.

Movement #6

- Slowly turn to the right and then back to center.
- Allow your low back and pelvis to move with the upper body.
- Move your knees a little in the direction you are turning.
- Breathe out as you turn.
- Let your eyes follow the movement of your nose.
- Breathe in as you come back to the center.

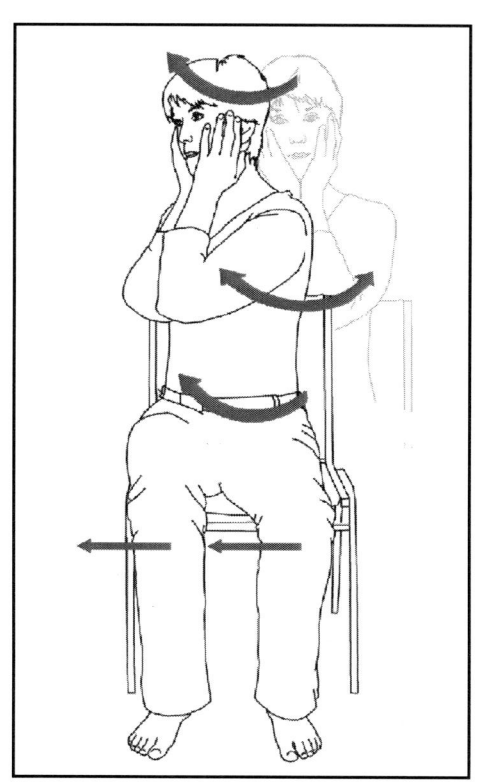

How does combining movements improve your ease in turning?

Sandra Bradshaw

Reference movement – notice the changes.

- Rest your hands on your thighs.
- Close your eyes and turn to the right and stay there.
- Open your eyes. Notice where you are relative to your reference point.

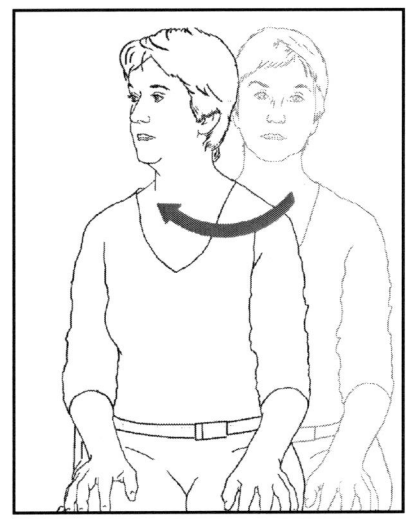

Notice what happened

- Did you spontaneously turn farther to the right?
- Is the movement easier now?
- You should now be aware of your whole body and how each part affects the movement.
- Did you spontaneously make use of the new strategies that improved your range and ease of movement?
- Turn to the other side and notice the difference.

In order for a movement to feel effortless, the whole body has to participate. Without full participation, the movement will be blocked and feel difficult. In this case, practice makes perfect! As you continue to work with this lesson, the new easier patterns of moving will become embedded in your brain and body, eventually becoming habitual.

Repeat the lesson on the other side.

Notes

Sandra Bradshaw

Lesson #7 – Comfortable Sitting

Develop Better Posture & Feel Comfortable

You may have noticed having good posture does not necessarily mean you feel comfortable. In that position you may even experience tight, achy muscles. Wouldn't it be nice to improve your posture and feel comfortable at the same time? Finding and maintaining a more neutral spine and pelvis, so your bones can support you, allows your muscles to be at rest. This makes sitting a more pleasurable experience.

This lesson will give you a strategy to help to alleviate discomfort. Your body will learn to find the support it requires to maintain good posture, yet be relaxed.

Time required to learn lesson
- 35 – 45 minutes

You will need
- A chair without arms and a firm level seat.

Take time to read the full lesson before you do it.

Reference movement – notice how you normally move.

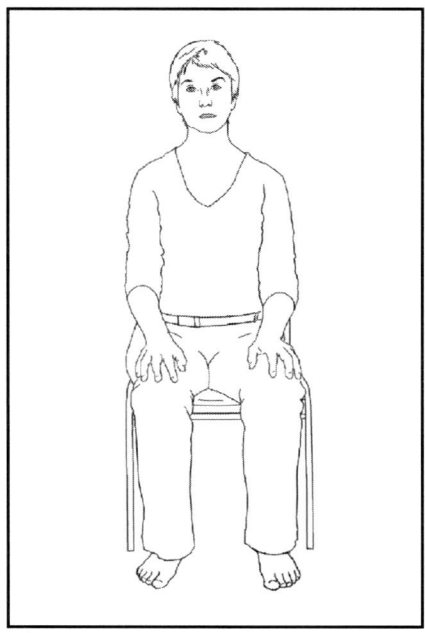

What to do

- Sit on your chair as you would normally sit.
- Don't do anything different.
- Make yourself comfortable.

What do you feel

- Are you slouching?
- Does your back feel rounded?
- Is your back rigidly straight?
- Notice any discomfort as you sit.

Typically, when sitting, a person is either slouched or rigidly straight. Neither of these positions is comfortable. They both contribute to tension, discomfort and/or pain. Make note of how you sit.

You will revisit your reference movement at the end of the lesson.

Sandra Bradshaw

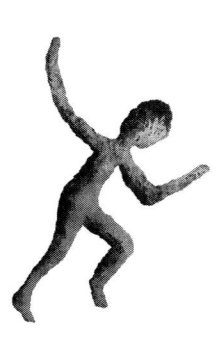

Tips for effortless movement:

Move slowly and make movements pleasurable.

Breathe naturally in an unhurried, easy manner.

Reduce effort to 50% of your capability.

Imagine a movement if doing it causes discomfort or pain.

Repeat each movement 3 or 4 times pausing between repetitions.

Starting Position

This is the starting position for all of the movements in this lesson.

- Sit toward the front of your chair.
- Feet are flat on the floor a comfortable distance apart (about a shoulder's width).
- Heels are positioned directly under your knees.
- Hands resting on your thighs.
- Eyes are looking out at the horizon.

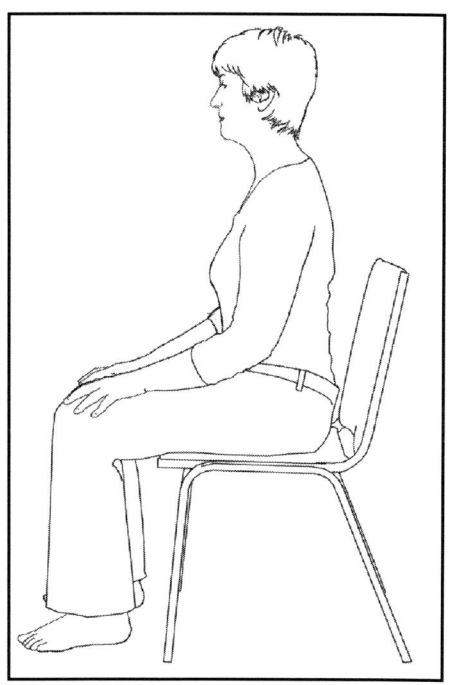

When your pelvis and feet are well connected to the surface they rest on, you are in a very stable position. Think of a three-legged stool; there is never a wobble even if the legs are different lengths. Ease of movement begins with a stable position, allowing you to move out of and back to your starting position smoothly.

Sit quietly. Release any tension you feel.

...ovement #1

- Start with your eyes looking towards the horizon.
- Slowly round your back.
- Let your chin drift down towards your chest and look towards your knees.
- Slowly return to your starting position.

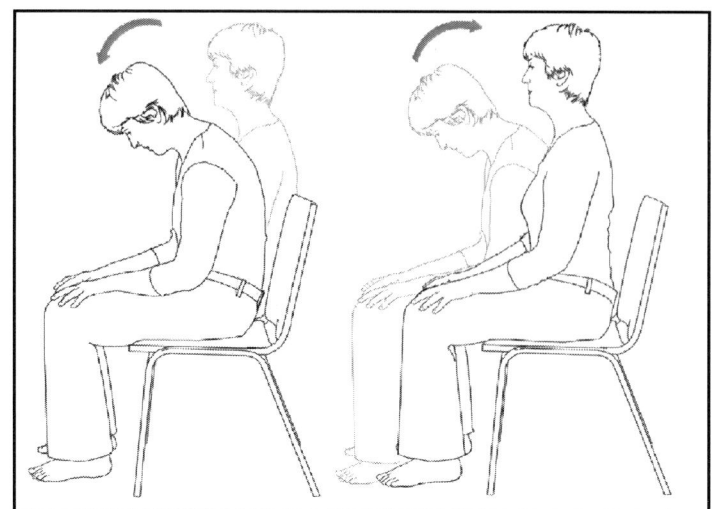

What do you feel

- Take note if you find this movement easy, or if it requires effort.

Movement #2

- Do the same movement but this time breathe out as you round your back and look down.
- Breathe in as you return to your original position.

What do you feel

- Note the difference in the quality of the movment when you change your breathing.

Pause for a few seconds between each repetition.

Movement #3

- Start with your eyes looking towards the horizon.
- Begin to arch your back.
- Let your chin move away from your chest and your eyes drift upwards.
- Slowly return everything to your starting position.

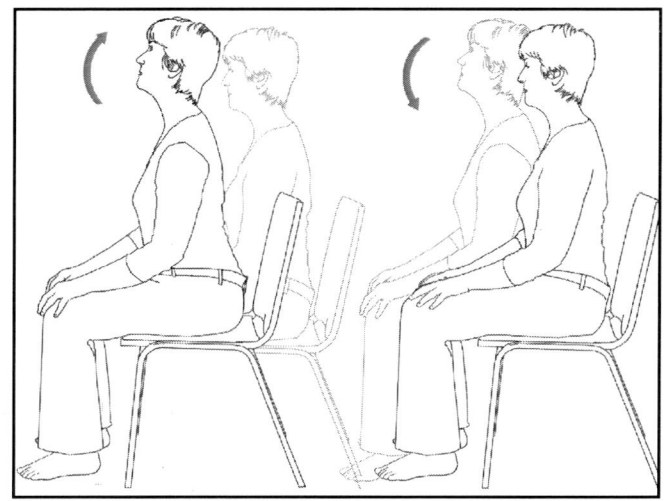

What do you feel

- Is this movement easier or more difficult than the previous movement of rounding your back?

Movement #4

- Continue with the same movement but alter your breathing.
- The first time, breathe in and arch your back and breathe out on the return.
- Next time breathe out when you arch your back and breathe in on the return.

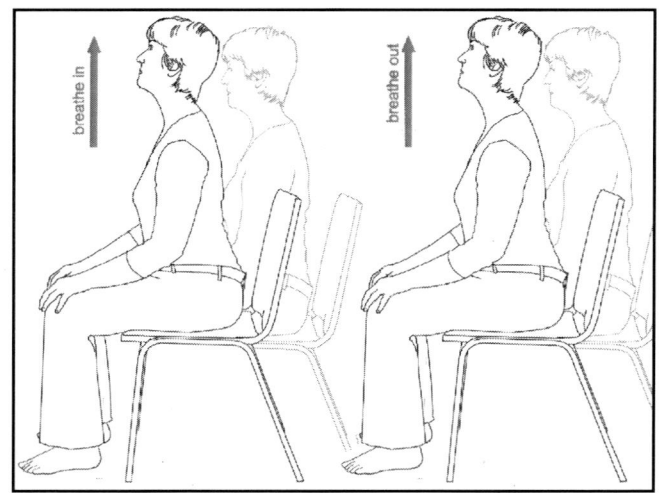

What do you feel

- Which way of breathing allows you to arch more easily?

It may feel more natural to breathe in and arch, but the range increases slightly, and the quality is softer if you breathe out as you arch and look up.

Allow your eyes to move up and down with your head.

You feel more when you do less.

Think of the lungs as balloons as shown in the drawing below. As the lungs deflate, if you are relaxed, you will automatically sink down and round your back. When you breathe in, your lungs will inflate, causing your trunk to unfold back to the upright position. Most people breathe in when they arch their back, thinking this will make the arching easier. What they don't notice is, by breathing in, arching is restricted and they need to push more to move in that direction. Deflating your lungs when you arch makes the movement easier.

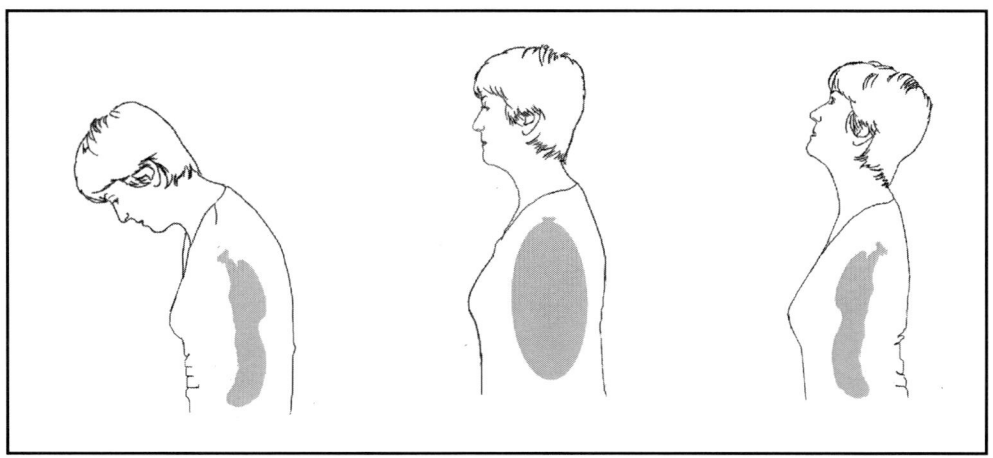

Movement #5
- Breathe out as you arch your back and look up.
- Breathe in as you return to your original position.

What do you feel
- How far can you move into the arch position when you breathe out as you arch?

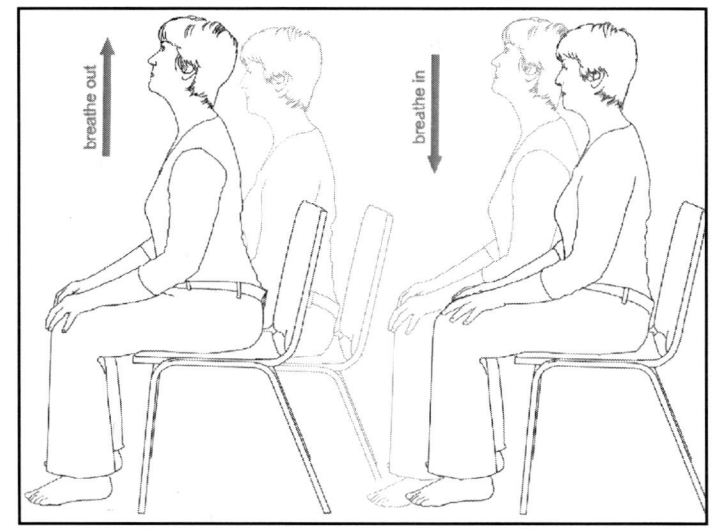

Your brain learns when you move slowly.

Sandra Bradshaw

Breathe naturally. Inhale and exhale gently.

Movement #6

- Combine the previous movements.

First

- Breathe in while you sit in your starting position.

Then

- Breathe out as you round your back. Drop your chin toward your chest.
- Breathe in as you return to your starting position.
- Breathe out as you arch your back. Move your chin away from your chest.
- Breathe in as you return to your starting position.

Note: Continue to do this sequence many times following the breathing pattern as you move from rounding to arching.

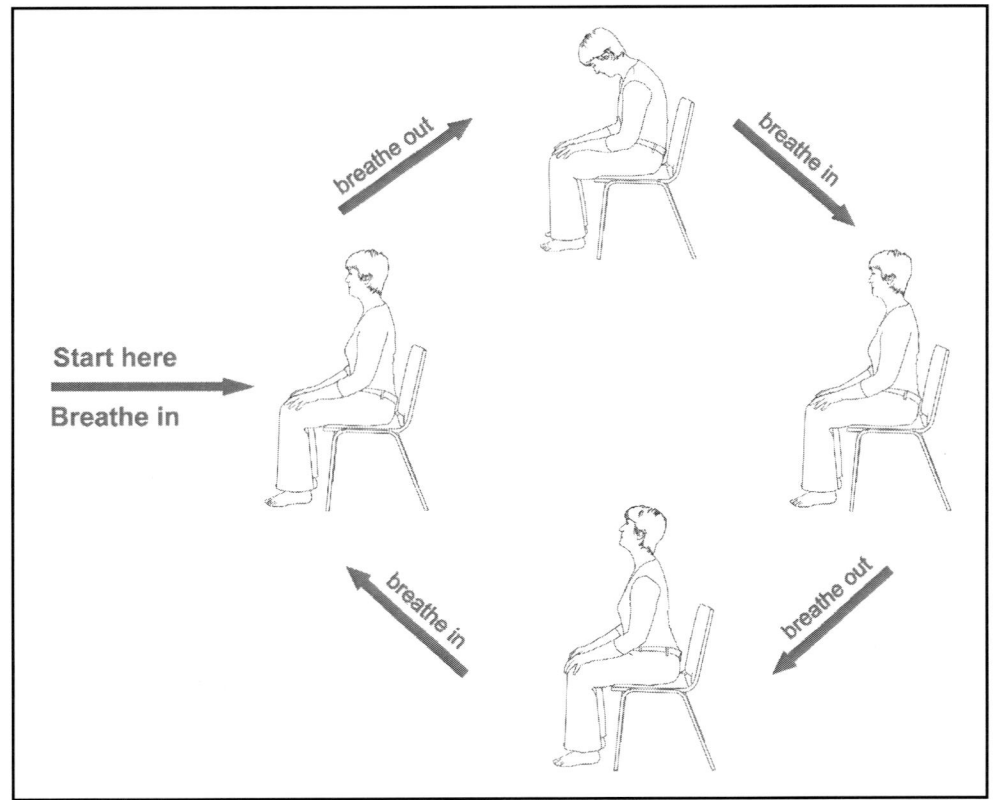

Decrease your effort. Move with your breath.

Movement #7

- Start in your normal position with your eyes looking at the horizon.
- Round your back and look up.
- Slowly return to your original position.
- Do this very slowly so that the two movements happen simultaneously.

What do you feel

- Are you able to continue breathing as you round and straighten your back?

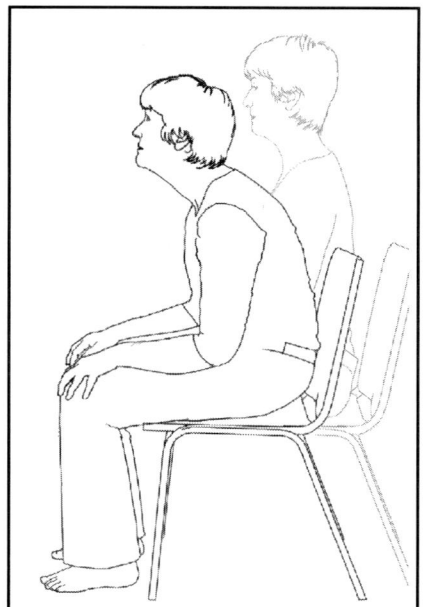

Movement #8

- Start in your normal position with your eyes looking towards the horizon.
- Arch your back and bring your chin toward your chest.
- Slowly return to your starting position.

What do you feel

- Are you able to continue breathing as you arch and straighten your back?

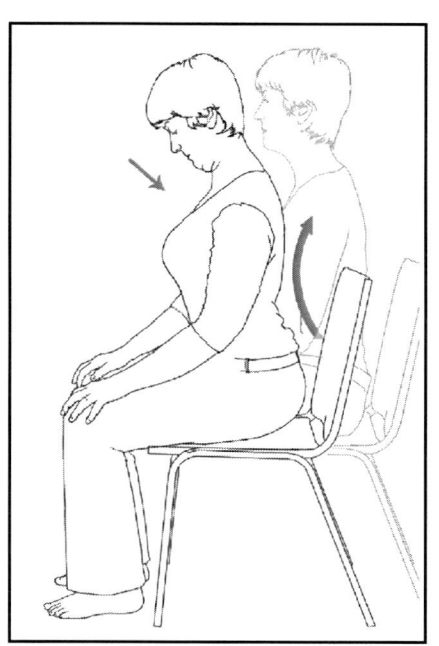

Rest between each movement instruction.

Movement #9

- Combine the previous two movements with your breathing.

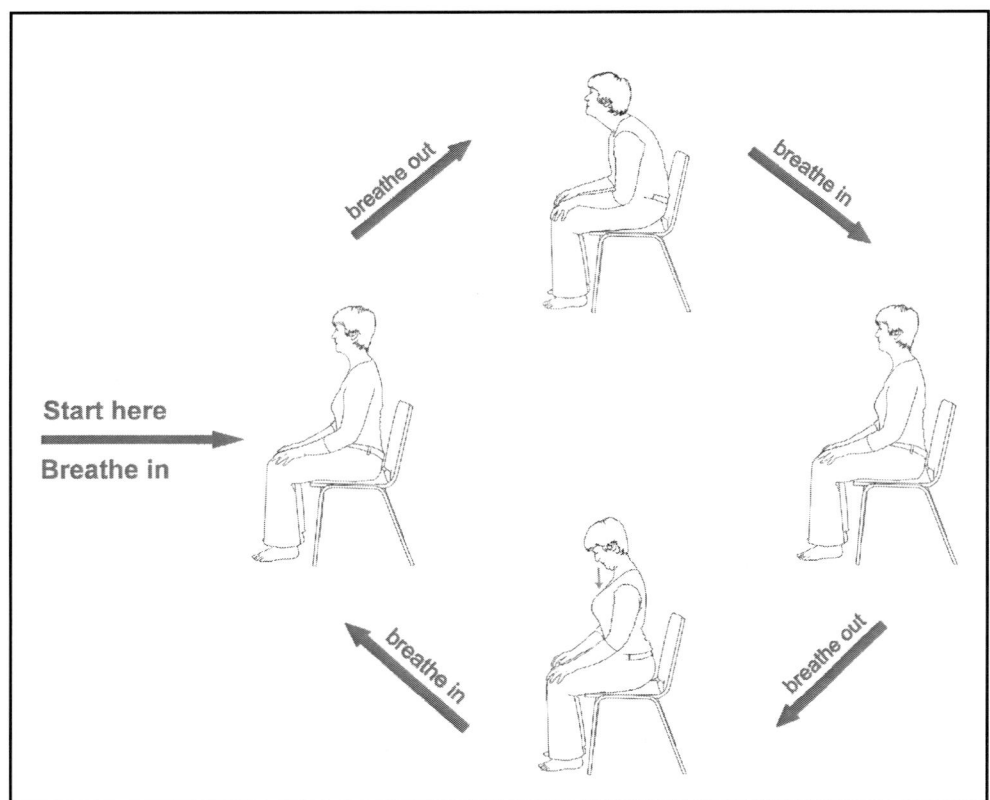

First

- Breathe in as you sit in your starting position.

Then

- Breathe out as you round your back. Move chin away from chest.
- Breathe in as you return to your starting position.
- Breathe out as you arch your back. Drop your chin towards your chest.
- Breathe in as you return to your starting position.

Note: Continue to repeat this sequence many times. Reduce your effort as you go. Continue to follow the breathing pattern as you round and arch your back.

Move your eyes in the same direction as your chin.

Reference movement – notice the changes.

- Sit on your chair as you would normally sit.
- Don't do anything different.
- Simply make yourself comfortable.
- Now remember how you were sitting before you started the lesson.

What do you feel

- Does your back feel different?
- Sit rigidly straight and notice how that feels.
- Sit in a slouched position and notice what that is like.
- Find the most comfortable position and notice where that is.

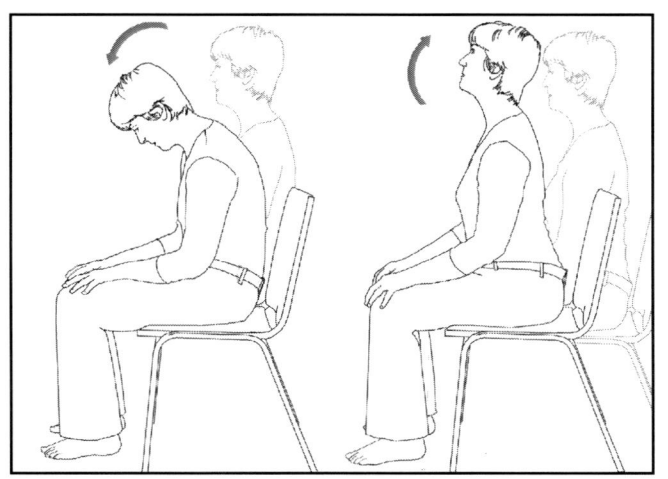

- Round and arch your back a few times.

What do you feel

- How is this different from the beginning?
- Are the movements easier and smoother than at the beginning?

Use this lesson any time your back gets tired.

Sandra Bradshaw

Something to consider.

The way you hold yourself when you sit, stand or lie down, is so deeply grooved into your brain it is difficult to change this postural habit.

You may have noticed that you will sit straighter or more symmetrically if you think about it, but if you don't pay attention you quickly go back to the old familiar pattern. Through these Awareness Through Movement (ATM) lessons you can get the brain to accept better alignment as your default.

Given the opportunity, your nervous system is attracted to movement that is pleasurable and easy. Your brain also pays attention to anything that is new and different. Therefore, if you do many different kinds of movements that feel good and are easy in ways that are fresh and different, the brain will eventually forget the habitual but uncomfortable pattern.

It will create a way of being that uses all of the functional, pleasurable information it has acquired.

Given a choice your body will choose pleasure over pain.

Notes

Sandra Bradshaw

Lesson #8 – Organize the Neck, Shoulders & Back

Novel Movements Change Patterns

Variety is the spice of life, particularly where movement is concerned. If you only have one way of doing something it limits your ability to move freely in any situation. When you extend your arms to reach for something on a shelf, hold the wheel of your vehicle, or write at your desk, it requires you move your arms away from your body. Yet, each activity calls for different arrangements of the bones, muscles and tissue.

In this lesson the variety of movements will enhance your ability to move your arms easily. Some of the movements may seem unrelated to reaching, but in the end, you may be surprised how variety changes outcome.

Time required to learn lesson
- 25 – 30 minutes

You will need
- A chair without arms and a firm level seat.
- A table or desk.

Take time to read the full lesson before you do it.

Reference movement – notice how you normally move.

What to do

- Stand in the middle of the floor with your feet a comfortable distance apart, and hands at your sides.
- Look up toward the ceiling and at the same time, reach up with your arms as if you were going to get something from a cupboard high above your head.
- Return to your starting position.
- This is your habitual way of moving.

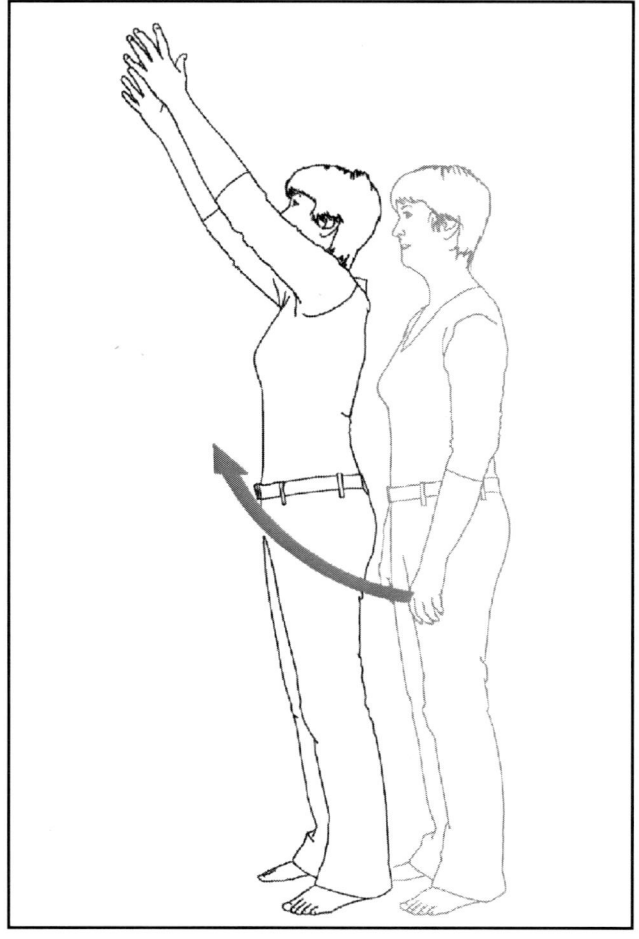

What do you feel

- How far are you able to reach?
- Make note if the reaching is easy or if it requires effort.

Remember what this felt like so that when you repeat the movement at the end of the lesson you will be able to feel the changes that occurred during the lesson.

You will revisit your reference movement at the end of the lesson.

Sandra Bradshaw

Tip reminders are at the top and bottom of each page.

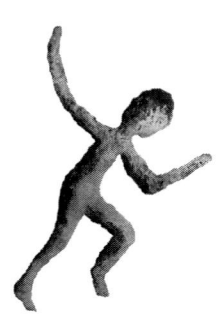

Tips for effortless movement:

Move slowly and make movements pleasurable.

Breathe naturally in an unhurried, easy manner.

Reduce effort to 50% of your capability.

Imagine a movement if doing it causes discomfort or pain.

Repeat each movement 3 or 4 times pausing between repetitions.

Your starting position

- Sit facing the desk.
- Have about a fist's width between your chest and the edge of the desk.
- Your pelvis is on the chair and your legs are free so they can move easily.
- Your feet are flat on the floor a comfortable distance apart (about a shoulder's width).

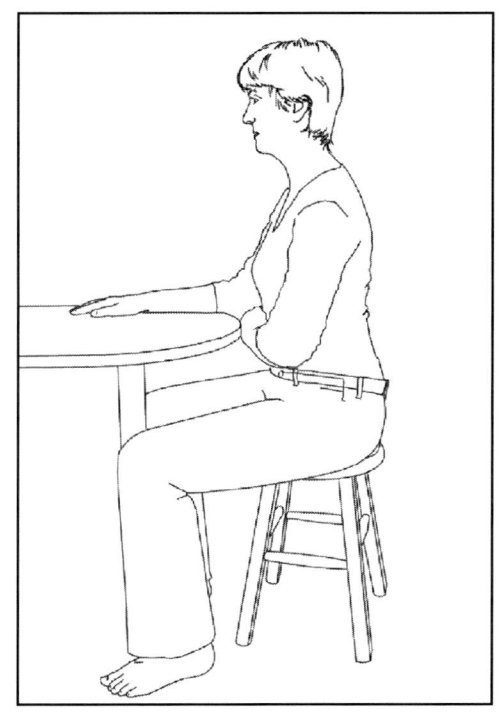

Note: You will be sitting in this position for the entire lesson. If your back feels tense it may help to put a small rolled up towel toward the back of your seat, tipping your pelvis forward. Another option would be to get up and walk around a little between each set of instructions to release tension.

Make sure you are comfortable before you start the lesson.

Repeat each set of instructions 3 or 4 times.

Movement #1

- Put the heels of your hands together.
- Cup your hands around your chin and cheeks.
- Put your elbows on the desk.
- Slide both elbows slowly away from you toward the back edge of the desk.
- Return to your starting position.

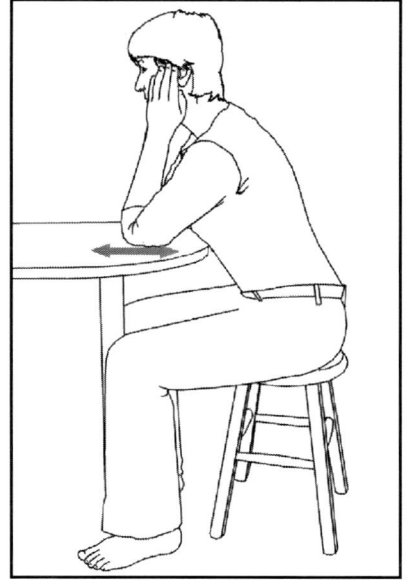

What do you feel

- Note how far are you able to slide your arms before your feel a strain.

Movement #2

- Put your hands around your chin and cheeks in the same fashion as before.
- Walk your elbows three or four small steps towards the back edge of the desk and then walk them back to the starting position.
- Allow more of yourself, including your chin to be involved in the movement.

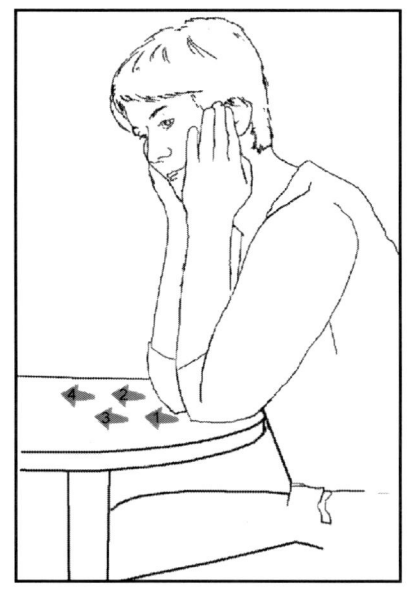

What do you feel

- Notice how your chin can turn from side to side as you alternate moving the elbows.

Only do what is easy. Don't strain.

Movement #3

- Keep your hands in the same position around your face.
- Lift one elbow in an arc out to the side and up towards the ceiling.
- Keep the other forearm perpendicular to the table.
- Your head will tip to the side as your right elbow lifts.

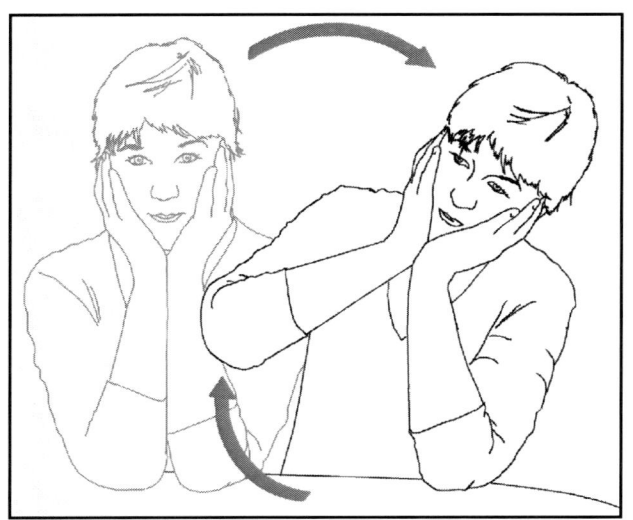

What do you feel

- Do you allow the wrist of the stationary arm to bend backwards as you lift the other elbow away from the table?

Movement #4

- Repeat the same movement on the other side.

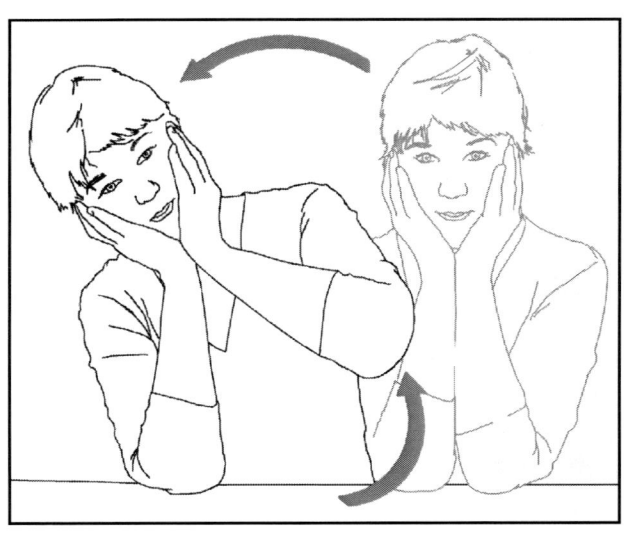

What do you feel

- How much effort does it take to move on this side?
- Do you breathe as you lift and lower your arm?

Less is more. Reduce your effort with each repetition.

Stay in the easy range as you move.

In order to develop equal ease and range on both sides you have to give the brain experiences that involve symmetry. To do this effectively, reduce the range on the easier side to match the range on the other side. Eventually the brain will stop identifying one side as less able and both sides will progress evenly.

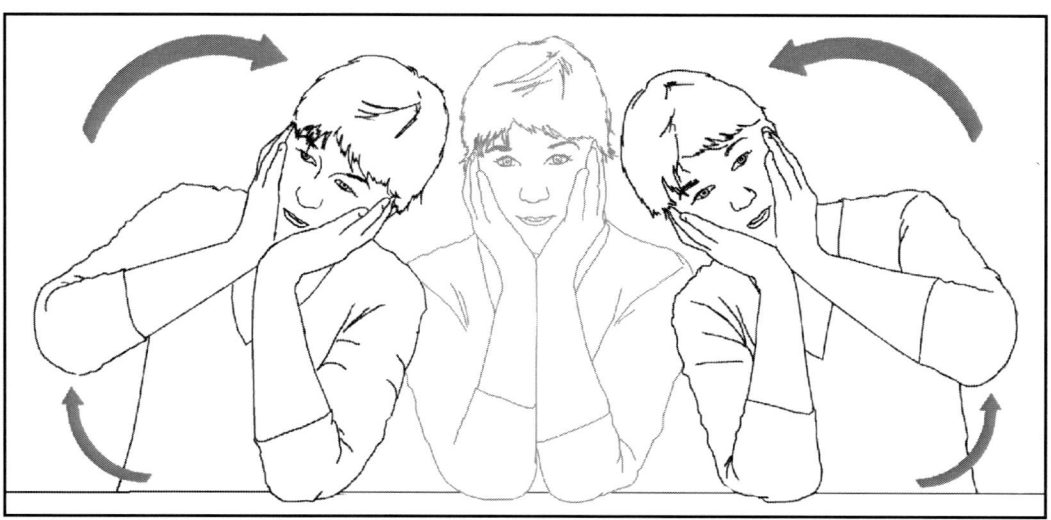

Movement #5

- Alternate lifting the elbows.
- Move slowly but continuously from side to side. Take at least 4 counts to lift the elbow and 4 counts to lower the elbow.
- If your range on one side is less than the other make the movements on both sides smaller so that you move symmetrically.

What do you feel

- Can you feel a new ease of movement?

Breathe. Holding the breath creates added tension.

Sandra Bradshaw

Reduce your effort as you move from side to side.

What you do with your eyes is an important, but usually overlooked aspect of movement. The eyes help direct movement and signal to the brain which muscles need to be activated and which muscles need to stay relaxed. If you fix the eyes on one spot, the brain thinks the body is going to stay still and holds the muscles in that position.

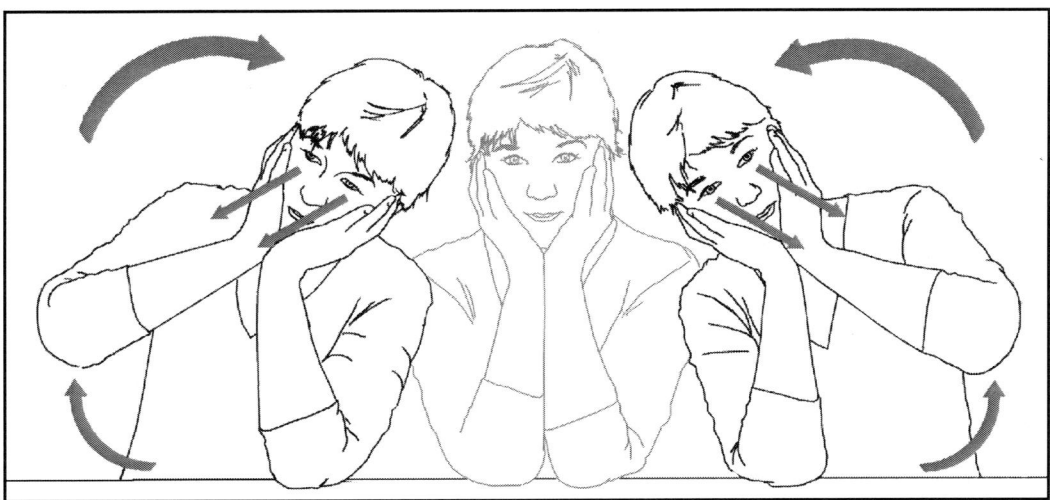

Movement #6

- Alternate lifting the elbows.
- Move slowly but continuously from side to side.
- Look in the direction of the elbow you are lifting. Repeat this a few times.
- Stare at something and don't move your eyes as you alternate the lifting.

What do you feel

- What is your range and quality of movement when your eyes follow your elbows?
- How does staring at one spot restrict the same movement?

Your eye movement should be gentle and easy.

Let your eyes move with the movement of your body.

Movement #7

- Put your right hand around your chin and cheek with your right elbow on the desk.
- Rest your left forearm on the desk with the fingers pointing forward.
- Make sure your elbows are about a shoulder width apart.
- Slide your right elbow towards your left elbow keeping your right hand on your chin and cheek.
- As your right elbow moves closer to the left elbow, allow your right ear to get nearer to the table.
- Your chin will move in an arc toward your left shoulder and your eyes will look toward your left arm.
- Allow your trunk to bend sideways as you turn.

What do you feel

- Where do you feel the bending in your back?
- Which side lengthens?
- Which side shortens?
- Notice if your pelvis shifts as you slide your elbow over.

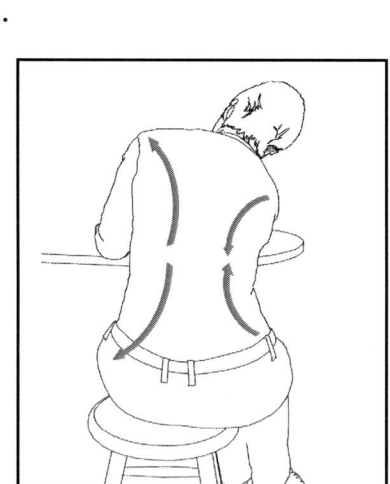

Note: Learning only happens when you notice what you do. When you are learning a new pattern of movement, do it slowly. Once you have learned it, you can do it at any speed you want.

Move slowly so you can notice what you are doing.

Sandra Bradshaw

Repeat each set of movements 3 or 4 times.

Movement #8

- Reverse the position of your hands.
- Repeat the last movement on the other side.

What do you feel

- Does the movement feel the same or different from the other side?
- Where do you feel the bending in your back?

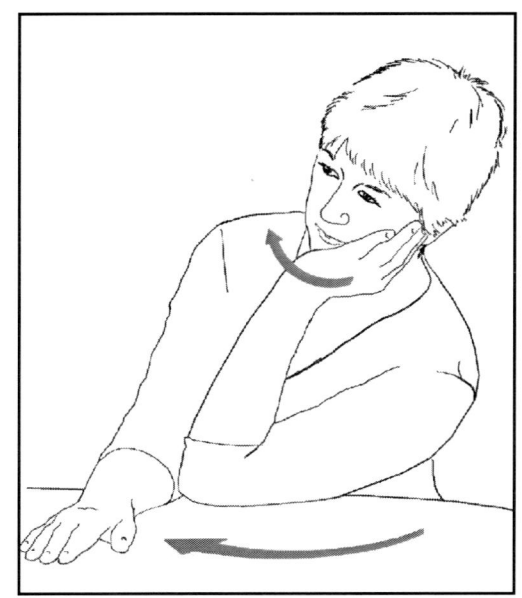

Movement #9

- Put your elbows on the table and cup your chin and cheeks with your hands.
- Keep one elbow stationary. This elbow will be the pivot point.
- Move the other elbow around the stationary elbow and back; you are drawing an arc on the surface of the desk.

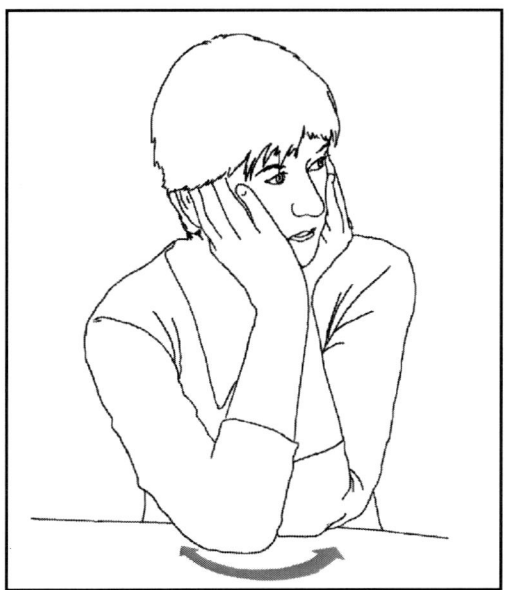

What do you feel

- How is your back moving as you move your elbow?

It's easier to be symmetrical if you keep your movements small.

Pause between each initiation of a movement.

Movement #10

- Do the same movement on the other side.

What do you feel

- Does the movement feel the same or different on this side?
- Where do you feel the bending and turning in your back?

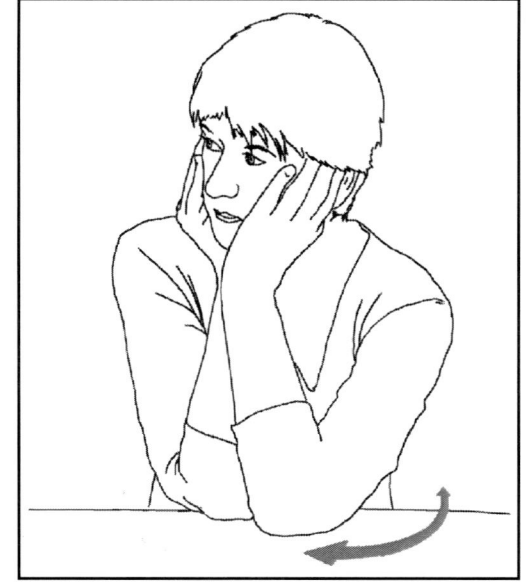

Movement #11

- Alternate; first making an arc with one elbow and then with the other.
- If your range of motion on one side is less than on the other, make the movements on both sides smaller so you move symmetrically.

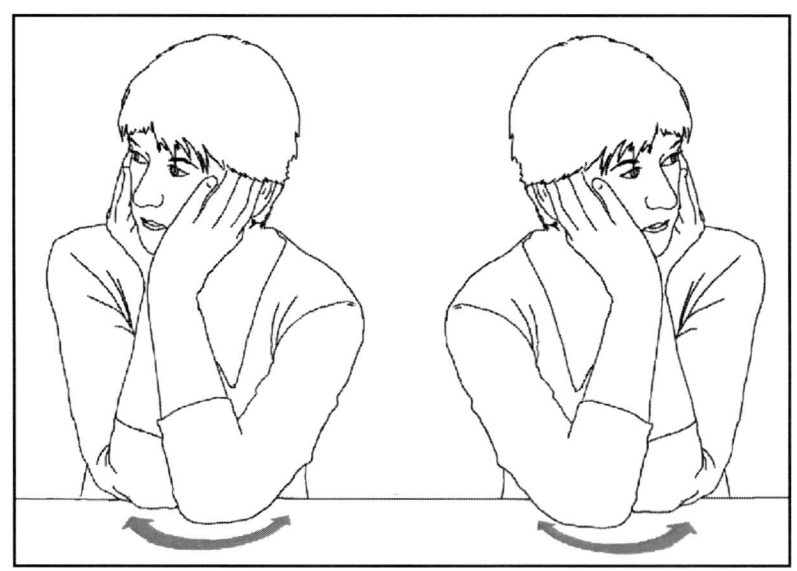

With each repetition of the movement, adjust for symmetry.

Sandra Bradshaw

Reference movement – notice the changes.

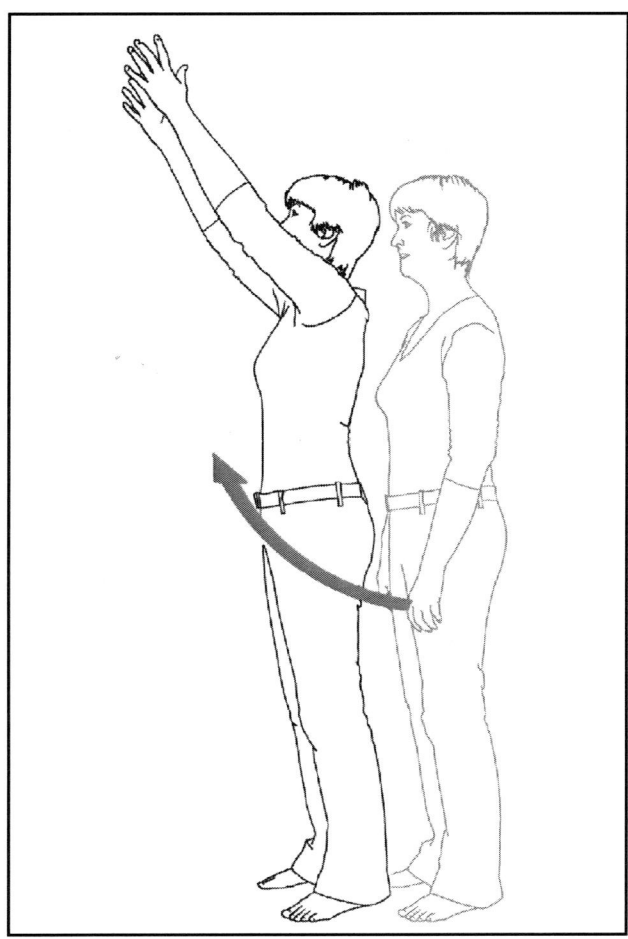

- Stand in the middle of the floor with your feet a comfortable distance apart, and hands at your sides.
- Look up toward the ceiling and at the same time, reach up with your arms as if you were going to get something from a cupboard high above your head. Return to your starting position.

What do you feel

- How does that movement feel now that you've completed the lesson?
- Has it changed from the first time you did it?
- Notice if you include your eyes in the movement.

Enjoy the changes you have created!

Notes

Sandra Bradshaw

Lesson #9 – An Easy Forward Bend

The Anti-Stretching Lesson

After years of dedicated stretching, your finger tips are still a long way from your feet! What prevents you from bending forward easily? The problem lies with the brain rather than the muscles. The brain is in charge of a finely tuned system of balance and counter-balance. When necessary, it will command specific muscles to tighten so you won't fall.

If tight muscles are a chronic problem, the solution is to provide your brain with an expanded repertoire of safe options allowing for easy forward bending. In this lesson you will bend forward in new ways without stretching.

With added information, the brain will reorganize the original movement and automatically give the signal to lengthen the required muscles. In the end, even if you don't touch your toes, you will get closer and feel more ease.

Time required to learn lesson
- 15 – 20 minutes

You will need
- A clear space in the center of the room where you can stand comfortably.

Take time to read the full lesson before you do it.

Reference movement – notice how you normally move.

What to do

- Stand in the middle of the floor with your feet a comfortable distance apart.
- Keep the muscles behind the knees soft and flexible.
- Do not lock your knees.
- Start with your eyes looking towards the horizon line.
- Without pushing yourself, bend forward as if to touch the floor.
- Only go as far as you can naturally and return to standing.

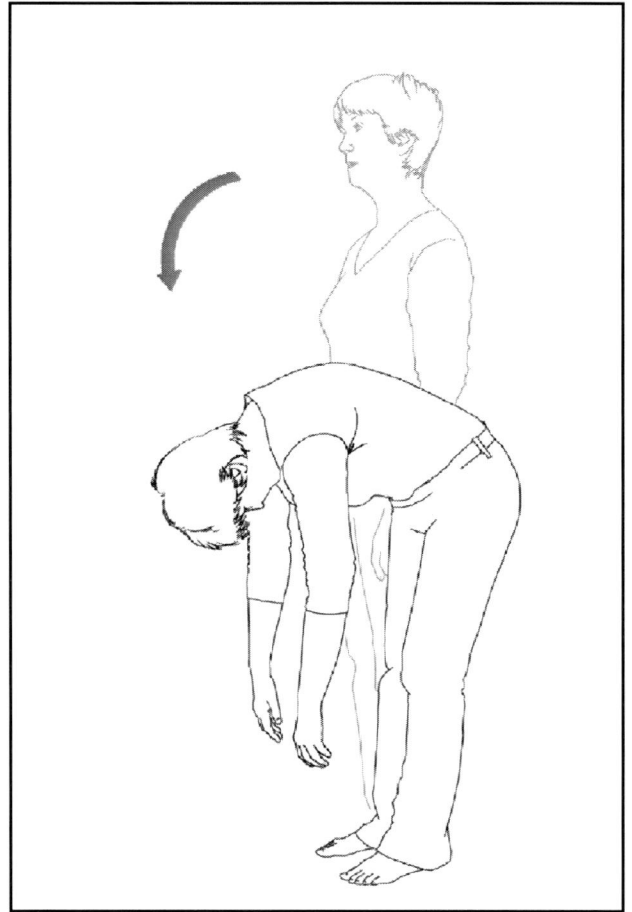

What do you feel

- When you are bent forward, notice where your hands are relative to the floor.
- Remember how far you were able to bend forward without effort.
- This is your reference point.

You will revisit your reference movement at the end of the lesson

Sandra Bradshaw

Effortless movement tips are at the top and bottom of each page.

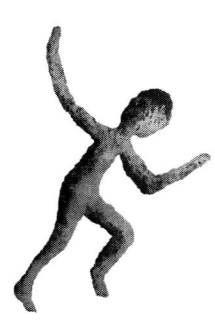

Tips for effortless movement:

Move slowly and make movements pleasurable.

Breathe naturally in an unhurried, easy manner.

Reduce effort to 50% of your capability.

Imagine a movement if doing it causes discomfort or pain.

Repeat each movement 3 or 4 times, pause between repetitions.

If you have restrictions in your back and you can't bend forward very far, that's okay. This isn't about straining toward the goal of getting your hands to the floor. It's about moving slow enough to notice how you are doing the movement and how it feels. Then you can improve the quality of the movement so it is smoother and easier.

Movement #1

- Start with your eyes looking at the horizon.
- Allow your chin to move gently towards your chest.
- Softly round your shoulders as you feel the weight of your arms pull you towards the ground.
- Release and round your back one vertebra at a time.
- Stop naturally and allow your head to hang without any strain or tension in the neck. Pause a moment.
- Reverse the movement and unroll yourself back to standing upright.

Repeat each set of movement instructions 3 or 4 times.

Pause between each initiation of a movement.

Have you ever noticed that when you concentrate on a new activity you hold your breath? Holding the breath increases tension in the body which creates resistance to movement.

Movement #2

- Breathe out as you begin your forward bend.
- Continue to exhale as you take yourself towards the floor.

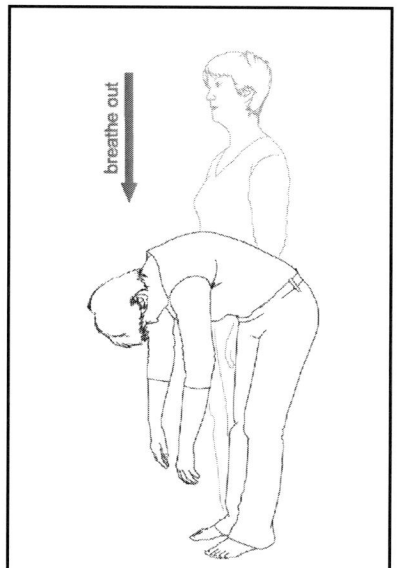

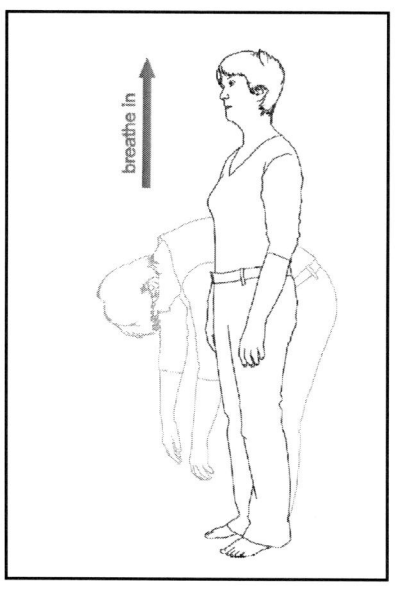

- Breathe in as you return to the standing position.
- Imagine that you are inflating two balloons in your chest and as they inflate it uprights your body.

What do you feel

- How does the quality of the movement change when breathing out as you fold forward, and then, breathing in as you stand straight?

Experiment

- Take in a full breath and hold it as you bend forward. Notice what that does to the range and ease of the movement.

Rest between each set of movement instructions.

Go slowly and let your body be pulled forward by gravity.

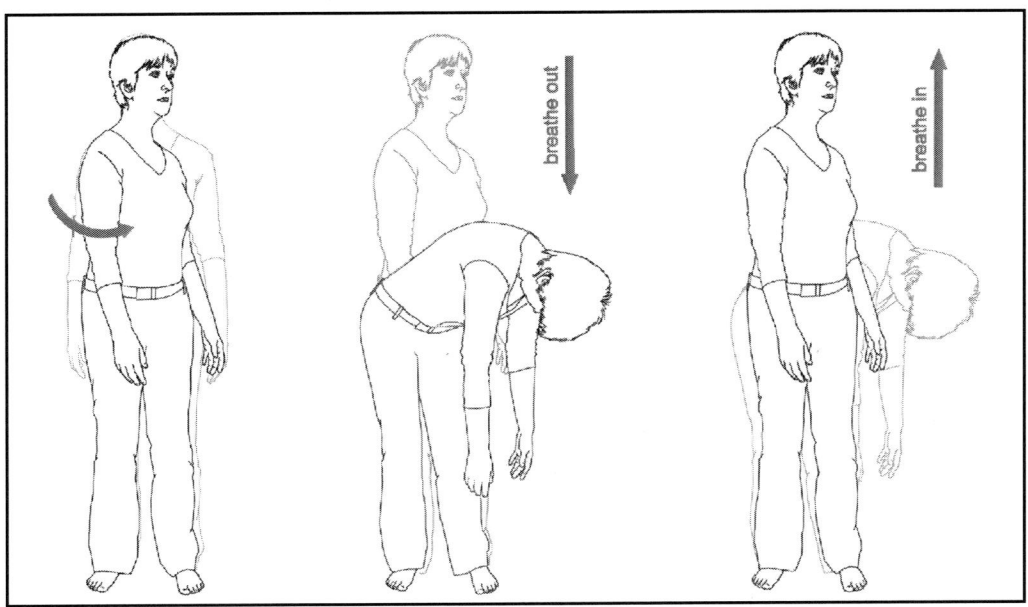

Movement #3

- Keep your feet pointed toward the front, but turn your body a few degrees to the left.
- Your body is now positioned over your left foot.
- Exhale as you gently drop your chin forward.
- Continue to exhale as your chest softens and your spine rounds.
- Keep the hands parallel to each other as you gently drop forward.
- Once you've reached your comfortable limit going down, inhale and allow the inflation of your lungs to help lift you back to standing.

In this turned position bending forward is deliberately restricted. Don't push yourself. Stop before it feels strained.

What do you feel

- Feel the tension diminish as you let your head hang passively and your arms dangle when you stop moving.

Make it easy. Decrease your effort with each repetition.

Remember to breathe with the movements.

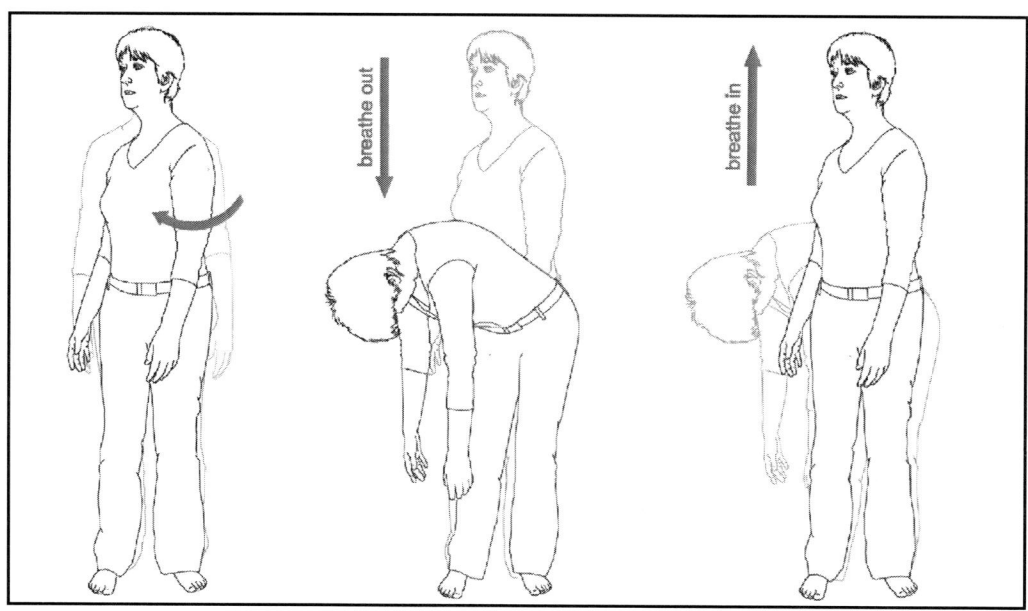

Movement #4

- Keep your feet pointed toward the front, but turn your body a few degrees to the right side.
- Your body is now oriented over your right foot.
- Exhale as you gently drop your chin forward.
- Continue to exhale as your chest softens and your spine rounds.
- Keep the hands parallel to each other as you gently drop forward.
- When you stop moving, stay there until air begins to fill your lungs.
- As you inhale allow the inflation of your lungs to help you come back to your upright position.

What do you feel

- Do you allow your head to hang passively and your arms to dangle when you stop moving?
- It should get easier with each repetition to coordinate your breathing with the bending and straightening of your back.

Allow your eyes to look in the direction you are moving.

Sandra Bradshaw

Reference movement – notice the changes.

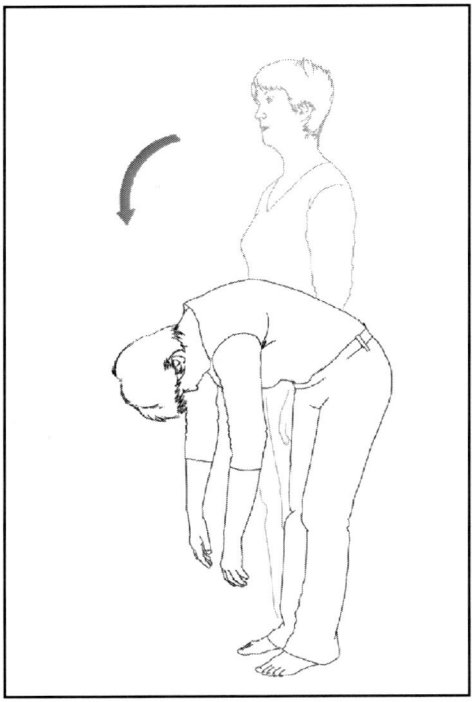

- Face toward the front, and without thinking about how you do it, move into a forward bend again.

What do you feel

- Remember your baseline movement and what it felt like.
- Where are your hands now in relation to the floor?
- What is the quality of the movement compared to the beginning?
- Are you able to move with less effort?
- Have you changed the way you breathe?
- Are you able to move with your breath?

Learning to easily bend forward improves your ability to stand upright without straining your lower back. As you practice this lesson and learn to work with gravity and your breath, you will find that you can surrender yourself to the ground and allow it to support you.

Improvement comes with awareness.

Notes

Sandra Bradshaw

Now What

You have just experienced a taste of the hundreds of Awareness Through Movement (ATM) lessons created by Moshe Feldenkrais. I urge you to contact your local Feldenkrais practitioner or go on line to my store at sandrabradshaw.com or the many other outlets that sell audio ATM lessons.

The lessons in this book are fully supported with audio lessons. For information about purchasing and downloading the audio versions go to sandrabradshaw.com. Click on Visit Our Store on the home page.

To experience a free audio lesson, visit sandrabradshaw.ca click on Store and Stuff, and then click Try Before You Buy.